THE CHILDREN'S SPORTS INJURIES HANDBOOK

A PRACTICAL GUIDE FOR PARENTS AND COACHES

Dr David Kennedy & Peter Fitzgerald

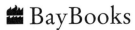
BayBooks
An imprint of HarperCollins*Publishers*

Dr David Kennedy is a Fellow of the Australian Sports Medicine Federation and has had a wide variety of experience in the treatment and research of sports injuries.

He was doctor-in-charge of the weightlifting competition at the 1988 Olympic Games in Seoul. He has been Consultant Medical Officer to the Victorian Cricket Association and was Medical Officer to the 1990 Australian Commonwealth Games team

Peter Fitzgerald is a Melbourne freelance writer who specialises in medical and consumer subjects for the popular market. He has written numerous books, including *You Can Sleep Soundly Every Night Without Drugs*, published by Bay Books.

The Children's Sports Injuries Handbook is a must for all parents and coaches.

A Bay Books Publication

Bay Books, an imprint of
HarperCollins*Publishers*
25 Ryde Road, Pymble, Sydney NSW 2073, Australia
31 View Road, Glenfield, Auckland 10, New Zealand

First published in Australia in 1988
Revised edition 1994

Text Copyright © David Kennedy with Peter Fitzgerald, 1988, 1994

This book is copyright.
Apart from any fair dealing for the purposes of private study, research, criticism or review, as permitted under the Copyright Act, no part may be reproduced by any process without written permission. Inquiries should be addressed to the publishers.

National Library of Australia
Cataloguing-in-Publication data:
   Kennedy, David, Dr.
     The children's sports injuries handbook.
     Rev. ed.
     ISBN 1 86378 131 5.
     1. Sports for children - Accidents and injuries. 2. Sports for children - Safety measures.
     3. Sports - Accidents and injuries. 4. Sports medicine. I. Fitzgerald, Peter, 1940- . II. Title.
     617.1027

Front cover: Fabio Nardo
Printed in Singapore
9 8 7 6 5 4 3 2 1
97 96 95 94

CONTENTS

Foreword 4

1 First steps for parents and coaches 5

2 Physical activity and the growing skeleton 20

3 Track and field 29

4 Football: australian rules, rugby league, rugby union and soccer 44

5 Bat and ball sports: cricket, baseball, softball and field hockey 58

6 Water Sports: swimming, surfing, water-skiing and sailing 68

7 BMX bike riding, skateboarding, rollerblading, horse riding, snow-skiing and ice skating 77

8 Racquet sports: tennis, squash and badminton 91

9 Netball and basketball 106

10 Strength sports: gymnastics and weightlifting 112

Ten golden rules for children's sport 121

Glossary 123

Index 126

Quick-find injury index 128

Foreword

This book can be considered essential reading for parents of sporting kids, coaches, teachers and also the medical and paramedical people involved in children's sport.

The authors have combined their respective talents to make a very important contribution to children's sport. With easy, non-clinical style, this book encourages us to read on as our understanding of children's sports medicine unfolds.

Colleagues and friends of David Kennedy respect him as a very dedicated doctor who obviously gains great satisfaction from helping sportspeople of all types and ages. His experience in sports medicine has been extensive; he has practised in the USA with professional football and baseball players, and worked with Australian Rules football teams, the Victorian cricket team and Olympic weightlifters. These experiences and his intense interest in younger sportspeople are testimony to his enthusiasm and commitment to our sporting community.

That Peter Fitzgerald's heart is well and truly in his work is exemplified by the fact that he once campaigned to popularise the use of helmets for child cyclists.

Among the many important messages to emerge from the book, two stand out. Firstly, children are not little adults — they must be treated specially as children. Secondly, parents can make a significant contribution to sports injury prevention in their children. This book tells us how to do both. We learn how injuries are related to maturation, types of sport, equipment and clothing, playing venues and climatic conditions. We do learn some new medical terms, but they are explained very carefully and a glossary makes it almost impossible to get lost during any description or explanation.

That this book is written to help kids stands out above all else. It is very clear that the experiences of fatherhood, as well as professional concerns, have inspired this fine publication.

Dr Richard Telford
THE AUSTRALIAN INSTITUTE OF SPORT
CANBERRA

CHAPTER 1

FIRST STEPS FOR PARENTS AND COACHES

Prevention of injury is the cornerstone of this entire book — be the sport a club, school or even a family activity. Prevention involves thorough preparation for the sport, knowing what to look for and erring on the side of commonsense and caution without ruining the fun of things. Children should equate sport with happiness, without the fear of getting hurt. You can quietly organise activities for children to unleash all their energy without them resenting an authoritarian heavy hand behind the scenes.

A vast number of children and teenagers are injured each year while playing sport — be it an organised sport or just for fun in the school playground, the local park, the street or an empty parking lot. Children just get carried away with their own immortality when attempting something just a little bit more daring than last time! Most mishaps need never happen. The experience of sports medical practitioners in Australia, the United States, Canada and Europe is that at least seven out of ten injuries to child athletes could have been avoided with advance knowledge of what part of their anatomy is the most vulnerable.

It must be stressed that sport is relatively safe. The benefits are enormous compared with the risk of injuries (which can be greatly minimised). It's my experience that the benefits for children of playing sport far outweigh the disadvantages of injury. Childhood is the time for athletic activity to provide the basis for long-term health, physical fitness and nutritional understanding.

Among physical and mental health professionals, there's no question that an appropriately-balanced athletic program is a positive factor in general physical and emotional development. We should strongly endorse such sports programs within our schools and communities.

However, as parents and coaches, we should be aware that all athletic events expose the participants to some degree of physical and emotional risk. The answer is to ensure maximum safety while permitting active participation.

This book for parents and coaches stresses self-help — with the proviso that you should seek medical attention for serious injuries or when in doubt about the nature of an injury.

In this book we have simplified medical and anatomical terms. The glossary at the back can be used as an easy reference or read in its own right as a summary of sports injury advice.

DO A FIRST AID COURSE

Knowledge of first aid is extremely important. Parents and coaches should consider doing one of the many excellent courses run by the Red Cross or St John Ambulance.

A senior first aid certificate can be completed through the St John Ambulance in two days at little cost.. From here, enthusiasts can undertake more advanced courses.

For further information on the St John Ambulance courses contact:

Adelaide	(08) 274 0444
Brisbane	(07) 252 3450
Hobart	(002) 23 7177
Melbourne	(03) 696 0000
Perth	(09) 334 1222
Darwin	(089) 27 9111
Canberra	(06) 282 2399
Sydney	(02) 212 1088

THE NATURE OF THE PROBLEM

Children are involved in about 40 per cent of all sports injuries. Two-thirds of these involve sprains, strains, contusions, abrasions and lacerations. Only about one in ten are fractures.

This isn't as bad as it may first sound because young children have tremendous resilience in overcoming injuries such as sprains, which would sideline a teenager or an adult for much longer.

The injury rate jumps as young players and athletes grow older. The competition is keener and the involvement is more physical. Older participants, especially boys, are heavier and stronger.

BOYS, GIRLS AND GROWTH SPURTS

Up to the age of ten, boys and girls are physically similar. The size of their bones and muscles is much the same and they have comparable athletic skills.

Girls start to mature from the age of ten. With adolescence and the start of menstruation, they experience hormonal changes which cause a growth spurt — a girl will grow as much as 10 to 12 cm (4 to 5 in) a year. This gradually ends somewhere between the ages of 14 and 16.

Seventy-five per cent of boys will start their growth spurt between the ages of 12 and 15 and the maturational growth period has usually ended by 18. Once the growth spurt slows, muscle mass increases. This usually occurs 6 to 12 months *after* the growth spurt ends, because bones and muscles grow at different rates.

As the muscle tissue develops, young adolescent boys and girls increase dramatically in strength and weight. Predictably, adolescents who mature earlier are more likely to succeed in most high school sports, particularly the contact sports such as various football codes and basketball.

There's considerable variation in individual maturation times. Boys

---

STOP

When in doubt seek medical attention.

generally experience their peak of skeletal growth at about 15 years of age, but some start at 13, while others don't complete this development until 17 or 18. This difference becomes significant when they engage in sporting activities.

Children whose physical and skeletal patterns mature early will be more powerful and better able to compete than late maturers. This is evident in all studies which have been made of adolescent athletes. Those who mature earlier are stronger and are thus more likely to succeed in primary school and secondary school athletics. Therefore, the problem is how to counsel late maturers about getting the best from their athletic and general sporting prowess. By the time they are 20 years of age, the late maturers will probably be taller and more skilled and stronger than the early maturers. However, while they are young, they shouldn't be mismatched (in the wrong sport or with the early maturers) in such a way as to cause them physical and emotional problems.

CHILDREN ARE NOT LITTLE ADULTS!

One of the most overlooked facts contributing to serious sports injuries is that children are children. They are not little adults. It is therefore essential that doctors, parents and coaches realise this and treat the injuries, and the problems that cause such injuries, accordingly.

CHOOSE SPORTS WISELY

Select sports and recreation activities wisely. This would go a long way towards preventing injuries in our youngsters. It is important to combine the child's ability and physical stature with a realistic and safe sporting achievement goal.

Assess athletic abilities carefully. Unrealistic expectations by coaches, parents and children are a major reason for many children withdrawing from physical education and sport.

Encourage participation by all. Handicapped children are frequently excused from sports participation for all the wrong reasons, when, in fact, they could benefit more from it than able-bodied children.

Monitor body development (muscle and bone growth). Physical mismatching is usually the result of indiscriminately grouping children by age rather than by physical characteristics and body development. These physical mismatches boost the injury rate by as much as 50 per cent — particularly in contact sports.

Check the selection process. Opponents of contact sports frequently cite the injury rate as a reason to drop a particular sport from the state (public) school curriculum. If, however, the selection methods were improved, injuries could be minimised. School administrators and sports coaches should look more carefully at the way children are selected for

There is considerable variation in individual maturation times.

A wise selection of sports helps prevent injuries.

Warming up maintains elasticity.

Correct technique is of the greatest importance.

participation in such sports. Only then will the injury rate in such contact sports fall dramatically.

Consider modifications and/or alternative sports. Game rules can be modified for different age groups to reduce the risk of injury. Too often, children and parents accept whatever team sports are available at school or in the community. Sometimes, they decide to just opt out. They don't realise there are numerous alternatives available to all children in both individual and team sports.

Reappraise your child and the sport. Conflict can be caused by the difference between the growth of the body and the technique of the sport itself. For example, a young gymnast with a light, pliant body can be disadvantaged once adolescent growth changes begin. Reappraisals may be necessary as the child grows and develops.

Use correct techniques. It's important to realise that some mechanical factors in a particular sports event, such as the specialised lifts in weightlifting, apply to all ages. Correct technique is therefore of the greatest importance.

THE MANAGEMENT OF YOUNG SPORTS PARTICIPANTS

General problems in the management of adolescents and young sports participants concern the planning of their training and general life. A long, successful sporting career can be enhanced by maintaining a balanced approach to training and fitness, with a good proportion of the different physiological components — speed, stamina, strength and mobility. All should get their fair share of attention. The supple, mobile young athlete is less likely to become a stiff, inactive person in later life.

THE ALL-IMPORTANT WARM-UP

Although children's natural elasticity makes soft-tissue injuries relatively mild and usually quick to heal, it's imperative that young athletes spend time warming-up to maintain this elasticity. A proper warm-up should include:

- General conditioning exercises that contribute to all aspects of the coming performance, particularly exercises promoting strength, power, speed and/or endurance.
- Exercises that reproduce the movements of the sport to be played, to prepare the body physically and mentally.
- Exercises such as gradual stretches, which will maintain flexibility and reduce the natural resistance and viscosity of the muscles, ligaments and other collagenous tissues.
- Exercises beginning gently and gradually building up in intensity.
- Exercises that are long and intense enough to raise deep body temperature and to break the sweat barrier.

STRETCHING

For maximum benefit and safety when stretching, follow these rules:
- Warm up before stretching.
- Never hold your breath when stretching: breathe slowly and deeply.
- Stretch before *and* after exercise.
- Stretch slowly and gently. Don't bounce or stretch rapidly.
- Stretch alternate muscle groups.
- Stretch muscles to the point of tension or discomfort but never pain.

Here is a stretching program for the major muscle groups used in most physical activities.

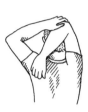 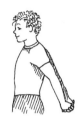 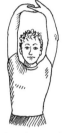 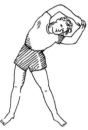

1 Stretch each arm for 15 seconds. Use your opposite hand to put pressure on the elbow.

2 Stretch for 15 seconds. Remain as upright as possible while moving arms away from the body.

3 Stretch up to the sky for 15 seconds.

4 Stretch to the side for 15 seconds each side. Do not lean forward while stretching.

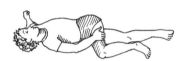 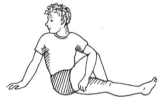

5 Keep your shoulders on the floor while holding your leg down with your opposite hand, for 20 seconds each side.

6 Draw both knees to the chest simultaneously. Pressure may be applied with the hands on the knees. Hold for 25 seconds.

7 Turn to the same side as bent leg. Apply pressure with your elbow on the knee and turn your head to the back.

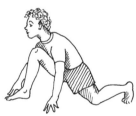 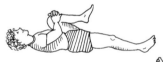 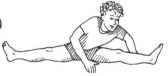

8 Aim to push the groin towards the floor while keeping your back leg relatively straight. Hold for 20 seconds each leg.

9 Draw one knee to the chest and apply pressure with your hand on the knee. Hold for 20 seconds.

10 During hamstring stretches, aim to put your chest on your thighs. Look forward, keeping your legs straight. Hold for 30 seconds each leg.

 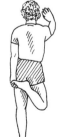 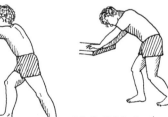

11 Sit with soles of the feet placed together and heels drawn as close to the body as possible. Look forward not down. Hold for 30 seconds.

12 Do not bend forward during this stretch. Draw the knee and hip back as far as possible. Hold for 15 seconds each leg.

13 & 14 During the calf stretches, keep the heels flat at all times. For stretch 14, bend the leg to stretch the soleus muscle. Hold for 30 seconds each leg.

First Steps

Dealing with stress

Motivation: Each athlete's ability and motivation should be assessed and realistic expectations defined. Motivation of the child in sport comes from peers as well as coaches and parents: this is positive feedback. Other children seem to be motivated by fear of failure. This group doesn't handle the stress of participation well.

Fatigue: This is a common problem with the young sports participant. The young adolescent needs adequate sleep and rest. This is a time for major growth, and this needs its own contribution of energy.

Balance: The development of talented young athletes often leads them to gain a distorted view of themselves. Sometimes this results in their paying less attention to their academic performance and personal growth. So never overlook the importance of achieving a balance between a youngster's academic, athletic and personal achievements.

Home environment: There are often many pressures at home, in today's environment of domestic problems and unemployment suddenly hitting families. Family breakdowns, separations and divorces also impose tremendous pressures on children.

Communication problems: Stress plays a big part in a wide range of common psychosomatic symptoms such as the stitch and vague abdominal pain or cramp. Sympathetic counselling, discussion and cooperation from parents, coaches and teachers can usually sort out such relatively simple problems as, for example, the conflict between schoolwork and examinations on the one hand and sporting pressures on the other.

Burnout: We have all heard and read about burnout with children or adolescents in sport. Burnout refers to the combination of physical and mental stress which has become more than the young athlete can handle. The normal methods of coping can't keep up with the increasing stress and eventually the young athlete cannot continue with the physical activities.

There are early warning signs of burnout which parents, coaches and health professionals should be watching for from time to time. These include sleeplessness, irritability, poor physical performances, recurring illness and/or injury, vague pains, lethargy, reduced motivation and fluctuating concentration span. Usually there is a combination of these symptoms: many athletes feel tired or experience pain associated with fatigue during normal training and competition.

Contribution: One of the great tragedies in Western nations is the tendency of adolescent sports participants to quit their sport when they leave school. This must largely be a reflection of unsatisfactory sporting achievements or the environment in which they participate. Parents, coaches and

Assess ability and motivation and have realistic expectations.

athletes can all contribute to improvements in the sporting arena.

Steps in Minimising Injury

Various European studies on young athletic participants identified at least 70 per cent of injuries as being preventable (for example: joint instability, muscle tightness or lack of flexibility, inadequate rehabilitation after injury and neglect of equipment or the rules). During the studies, correction of these factors reduced the injury rate by 75 per cent, compared with the other, uncorrected teams.

The injury rate can be substantially reduced by proper preventive measures:

- Select youngsters for sports on a more scientific basis: according to their anatomical and physiological suitability. Unfortunately, some parents and coaches have such a rush of blood to the head that they seem incapable of being objective about physical criteria such as body size and development.
- Analyse the individual's sporting style. The prowess of individual participants will depend largely on the correction of their faults. This doesn't require expert knowledge of all sports by school administrators, parents, coaches and doctors. Rather, it calls for being alert for mismatching: putting the individual in the wrong sport.
- Carefully select and fit all sporting gear and equipment. Your aim should always be to buy the best possible equipment within your budget — and then correctly wear or use it.
- The continued improvement of all types of playing surfaces, facilities and athletic equipment. This is a particularly important factor. Also, careful treatment and consideration of the injured athlete may prevent further injury and ensure that permanent problems don't develop.
- Spending time becoming familiar with the rules and fundamentals of the sporting activity. Lack of familiarity can cause sporting problems and stress, making children and young adolescents awkward and accident-prone.
- Pre-condition young athletes to develop strength, endurance, flexibility and speed so they can cope with hazardous situations. A tackle, or a push from the side, may move a particular joint beyond its limit, resulting in an injury to the capsule, ligament or adjacent muscle and tendon. Therefore, calisthenics and mobility exercises are extremely important in preparing for sporting activities. The increase in flexibility and range of joint movement, coupled with the strengthening of supporting muscles, enables the young participant to withstand more severe strain, impact and twisting than previously.

Good conditioning, gear and equipment are essential.

At least 70 per cent of injuries are preventable.

High sugar drinks can make you feel sick, give you stomach cramps or even diarrhoea.

Extra protein will not produce an increase in muscle size.

Some Common Myths about Food and Nutrition in Sport

Myth: A high energy drink prior to a game will give me heaps of energy.
Answer: It will for a short time but the high sugar intake sends signals to the body (by increasing blood levels of insulin) to use more sugar. The glycogen stores are used up more quickly and your stamina decreases. High sugar drinks can make you feel sick, give you stomach cramps or even diarrhoea.

Myth: If I'm sweating a lot, I need to take salt tablets.
Answer: You are losing some salt in your sweat but you are losing a lot of water with the salt. If you take salt tablets, you only increase significantly the water you are losing. This results in increasing dehydration, which can lead to stomach cramps, muscle cramps, dizziness and even vomiting. If you are sweating a lot, drink pure water, not salt tablets. If you know it's going to be hot before an activity, prehydrate with water two to three hours before the activity.

Myth: Extra protein will build up my muscles.
Answer: Extra protein will not produce an increase in muscle size. Muscles will grow only after they have been stimulated by weight-bearing exercise such as weight training. Your normal well-balanced diet will provide enough protein and there is no need for protein supplements. You should eat in your diet about 50 to 60 per cent carbohydrates, 30 to 35 per cent protein and 5 to 10 per cent fat. If you eat too much protein or fat instead of carbohydrates, your glycogen stores will not be filled and you will have less performance and stamina. Protein and fat are inefficient sources of energy.

Myth: Vitamins provide extra energy.
Answer: Vitamins and minerals cannot be used as an energy source. They do, however, take part in chemical reactions in the body which release energy from carbohydrate, protein and fat. A balanced diet will provide all the vitamins and minerals you need.

The Pre-game Meal

By the morning of a game, your glycogen stores should be very high if you have been eating a high carbohydrate meal each day. It is a good idea to have a high carbohydrate meal two to three hours before a game if you can because it will:

1 Reduce hunger and lightheadedness during the game.
2 Top up the glycogen stores so that they will be at a maximum level.

There are several things to consider with the pre-game meal.

TIMING

Preferably eat the meal two to three hours before the game, to allow insulin levels to return to normal before the game begins. Remember, eating or drinking a high sugar meal within the hour before a game increases insulin in the body, resulting in the glucose being used more rapidly and reducing available energy sources.

Eating a meal too close to a game can cause stomach cramps and may make you ill, especially if you are tense or nervous about the game.

SIZE AND CONTENT

The meal should be light, meaning low in fat and protein but high in carbohydrate, and not a large serving. It should be a familiar and enjoyable meal that holds no hidden surprises. Avoid foods that give you indigestion or increased wind.

ALTERNATIVES

If you are unable to have a meal two to three hours before a game, drink a diluted unsweetened fruit juice or skim milk (about a cup) no later than 30 minutes before the game as a good substitute. A high carbohydrate meal the evening before the game will also help (for example, pasta or rice).

PRE-GAME FOOD TIPS

- Eat foods high in carbohydrate to top up muscle energy stores.
- Go for low-fat foods for quick digestion.
- Eat two to four hours before exercise to allow time for digestion.
- Feel comfortable, not full.

HIGH CARBOHYDRATE MEALS

- Spaghetti on toast.
- Toasted baked bean sandwich.
- Toast, honey and fruit juice.
- Fruit smoothie, such as low-fat milk, yoghurt and banana blended.
- Pasta with vegetable sauce.
- Stir-fried vegetables with steamed rice.
- Baked potato stuffed with baked beans.
- Breakfast cereal and low-fat milk topped with fresh fruit.

EXAMPLES OF PRE-GAME MEAL FOODS

- Packet breakfast cereals
- Porridge
- Fruits and fruit juice
- Bread, toast, rolls
- Crumpets
- Muffins
- Biscuits
- Scones
- Pancakes
- Pasta or noodles

Drink a glass of water in the last 30 minutes before the game. This helps stop you becoming dehydrated during the game.

DURING THE GAME

If you have prepared before the game with a high carbohydrate diet and pre-game meal then you will have

Eating a meal too close to a game can cause stomach cramps.

Drink a glass of water in the last 30 minutes before the game.

The most important thing to drink during the game is water.

sufficient energy and will not need to drink sugar drinks during the game. The most important thing to drink during the game is *water*.

After the Game

You don't need to replace lost energy after the game with a sweet drink. Your normal high carbohydrate meal pattern will restore your glycogen stores. Water is all you need after a game to rehydrate yourself.

Understanding Equipment

Strapping for prevention, and strapping an injury

It's a common fallacy that strapping can protect against injury, regardless of the circumstances. It should always be remembered that protective devices have their limitations and that, occasionally, they may even increase the injury risk of some sports.

Strapping cannot prevent injury.

If you're dealing with a young player who has injured a particular joint, and you're deciding whether to apply a bandage to that joint to give mechanical support or protection to enable a return to the sporting activity, you must make the decision using sound anatomical principles.

The most fundamental questions to consider are: what is the problem and how will that joint be used after the injury?

For example, if you have just pulled a muscle, which has now become swollen because of bleeding, and isn't fit to support normal movements, you should *never* try to perform those normal movements with the assistance of strapping or bandages applied to the injured muscle. No amount of strapping will be safe.

It's bad medicine and psychologically unsound to allow a convalescing young player to resume attempts to play until he, or she, is anatomically sound. That is, the injury has to heal with a resumption of full function to the area. Usually, when this has occurred, the participant doesn't need help from bandages or non-stretch tape.

Non-stretch tape

There's considerable value in using non-stretch tape on joints. It does two things:

1 It may give a little mechanical support to ligament structures.
Example: A classic example is the U-shaped stirrup applied to an ankle joint following a sprain. The stirrup allows the hinge movement of the ankle to occur with minimal restriction and adds support to the ligaments on either side of the ankle during twisting and turning movements.

2 It may enhance the joint's awareness of its surrounding circumstances (known as 'proprioception').
Example: When the foot is planted on the ground and moves slightly,

this nervous awareness of the joint sends messages to the brain which, in turn, sends a message to the muscles which support that particular joint. This enhances the joint's functional stability when load-bearing forces are applied.

CATEGORISING SPORTS INJURIES

Sports injuries can be divided into two kinds: trauma injuries and overuse injuries.

Trauma injuries are those involving contact with other players, equipment or other obstacles during participation in a particular sporting activity.

Overuse injuries, which account for about one-third of all reported injuries, are simply due to the locomotor system — that is bones, joints and muscles — showing dynamic symptoms of stress. In other words, an athlete may excessively stress either a muscle or a capsule lining of a joint in a sporting activity by using it constantly and repetitively over a long period or repetitively and intensively over a short period. This constant, repetitive use causes those tissues to break down and malfunction, which means limitations to certain movements.

Overuse injuries can vary from muscle stiffness to the stretching of a tendon or ligament due to unaccustomed or prolonged repetitive exercise. They include injuries involving the soft tissues and injuries involving the bone itself, including the classic stress fracture.

A stress fracture is caused by repetitive stress to a bone, resulting in the breakdown of the bone's normal structure. This is in contrast to a fracture that occurs because of trauma — usually an intense force applied to the bone which results in the immediate breakdown of the architectural structure.

The essential point about overuse injuries is that no one but the participant is responsible for the overuse injury and that this breakdown — whether it involves muscles, tendons, ligaments or bones — relates only to the mechanical movements undertaken.

The age pattern of sport is gradually changing so that many young children and adolescents are today being subjected to loads far greater than those once thought acceptable, in terms of the mechanics of movement involving particular bone and muscle structures.

Ambitious parents and coaches don't easily see why their children should be 'second rate'. They simply don't understand the many mechanical factors operating in different sports. These parents and coaches often don't understand that the risks their children take in certain sports could be sensibly minimised without lessening the enjoyment and the chance of winning.

Understanding the varying

Sports injuries can be divided into two kinds: trauma injuries and overuse injuries.

Risks can be minimised without lessening the enjoyment of the sport or the chance of winning.

First Steps 15

See a doctor with any injury which causes severe pain, hasn't healed within three weeks or is infected.

mechanical stresses which are applied to the locomotor system in different sports, and understanding how preventive measures can help avoid such injuries, are two of the keys to successful management of children in sport.

Coping with Injury: RICE

The cornerstone of all sports injury treatment is RICE. This is the most important immediate treatment for all athletic injuries, whether the child has pulled a muscle from a strained ligament or broken a bone. The letters in the acronym stand for Rest, Ice, Compression, and Elevation.

Rest is essential, because continued exercise or extended physical activity could increase the length of time the injury persists. Stop using the injured part the minute that part is hurt. Use a sling or crutches if necessary.

Ice decreases the bleeding from the injured blood vessels by causing them to contract. The more blood that collects in a wound, the longer it takes to heal.

Compression limits swelling which, if uncontrolled, could slow down healing. Following damage to a tissue, blood and fluid from the surrounding tissues bleed into the damaged area and distend the tissue. That's all swelling is. Swelling can be useful in some instances, particularly if the skin is broken and the area has become infected. Antibodies then collect in the swelling to kill the germs. But, if the skin hasn't been broken, antibodies may not be necessary and the swelling can delay healing.

Elevation of the injured area to above the level of the heart helps the blood return to the heart by using gravity to help drain excess fluid from the damaged area.

When to See a Doctor

If you are concerned about the injury and are unsure about whether the child should see a doctor, I recommend these guidelines:

Pain. Any injury which causes severe pain should be seen by a doctor because pain is nature saying that something is seriously amiss. When it's severe, you should 'listen'. Also, if the pain in a bone or joint persists for more than two weeks, then these tissues are the ones in which the most serious injuries have occurred.

Joint injuries. All joint injuries should be seen by a doctor. This also goes for any injuries which haven't healed within two weeks. They should be checked for structural abnormalities. Injuries to a joint involve damage to a capsule and possibly ligaments. If not treated promptly, these injuries have the potential to become permanent and cause significant future problems.

RICE:
STEP-BY-STEP PROCEDURES

Swelling usually starts within seconds of an injury, so start RICE immediately. Don't wait for a doctor's advice.

1 Rest the injured part completely.

2 Place a wet towel over the injured area. Apply ice in the form of an ice pack, ice chips or ice cubes in a wet towel. Never apply the ice directly to the skin or in a plastic ice pack, because it can cause the skin to burn and become painful.

3 For compression, wrap an elastic bandage firmly over the ice around the injured part. Be careful not to wrap the area so tightly that you cut off the blood supply. The signs of a shut-off blood supply are numbness, cramping and further pain. If any of these occur, immediately unwrap the injured area. Otherwise, leave the ice pack and the bandage in place for approximately 30 minutes.

4 Elevate the injured area so that it is above the level of the heart.

5 Next, to allow the skin to become warm and the blood to recirculate, unwrap the area for 15 minutes. Repeat this procedure every three to four hours. If the area continues to swell, or pain increases, immediately check with a doctor (if you haven't already done so).

6 With a severe injury, you can follow the RICE program for 48 to 72 hours, having consulted your doctor. Further treatment depends on the type of tissue which has been injured.

The cornerstone of all sports injury treatment is RICE. Rest, Ice, Compression, and Elevation.

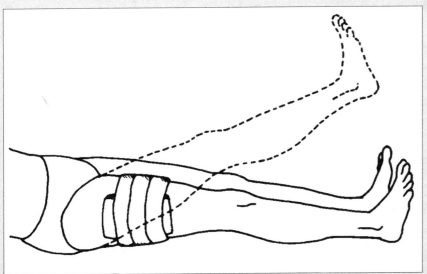

RICE, the cornerstone of early treatment for muscle and joint injuries.

> *If you're unsure about whether a doctor should be seen, err on the side of caution.*

Any joint injury should be immobilised until seen by a doctor. **Lost function**. If the child cannot move a limb or a joint (such as an ankle or a finger) the injury should be assessed a soon as possible.
Infection. Any injury which appears to be infected (manifested by pus, skin discolouration, swollen lymph nodes or fever) can lead to serious complications if uncontrolled. Antibiotics generally, bring quick relief.

Please note, however, that every injury is an individual event and every situation is unique. If you're unsure about whether a doctor should be seen, err on the side of caution. Use commonsense but don't take risks with someone else's health.

How Long will it Take to Recover?

The golden rule in orthopaedics is three days, three weeks or three months. That was almost holy writ in my medical training. But I've learned through hard experience that life and medicine are not that simple. The doctor and the patient should always expect the unexpected!

Healing time mainly depends on blood supply because the blood brings the elements necessary for the healing to occur:
- **Nutrients.** Think of the injury as a remodelling job. Nutrients are the building materials for healing.
- **Oxygen.** This is the energy source for the healing project. I tell my patients that you can't have fire without oxygen. Similarly, the body can't heal without oxygen.
- **Inflammatory cells.** These are the workers in the healing process. They carry away the old blood and the dead tissue. They also fight off infection by assembling the building blocks. Unfortunately, the best they can do is a slick patch-up job. Most body tissue, except the liver, heals with scar tissue. The larger the injury, the bigger the scar. The body never really totally forgets an injury.

When can Sport be Resumed?

Here are my guidelines:
- If the injured area hurts at rest, it shouldn't be exercised.
- As soon as the injured part doesn't hurt at rest, it may be exercised minimally. That means *slowly*. If the pain resumes, stop exercising. Listen to the body signals!
- As soon as the exercise can be handled without pain, increase the intensity and the duration of the exercise program gradually. Expect a little aching. But remember to stop *immediately* sharp pain starts.

When recovering from any athletic injury, it's important to maintain cardiovascular fitness. Thus, if a child has an injured ankle, encourage him/her to try a sport that doesn't require strenuous use of the ankle. For example, try swimming. If it is a wrist injury, try bicycling. It only

> *If the pain resumes, stop exercising. Listen to the body signals!*

takes about six weeks to lose cardio-vascular endurance. Any exercise will be of more benefit than resting in bed or sitting in a warm bath.

If a child doesn't quickly rehabilitate after an injury, muscles will remain in a weakened condition. Even if the child returns to full sports activity, the muscles will remain weak and he/she will subconsciously favour the injured limb.

The body will simply not feel right until full strength has returned. Also, a child will be very vulnerable to re-injury. In a weakened condition, an injured part simply cannot protect itself against the stress of sports participation. So make sure the injured part is fully healed before returning to the sporting activity that caused the injury in the first place.

Make sure the injured part is fully healed before returning to the sporting activity that caused the injury.

WHEN SHOULD ASPIRIN BE USED?

Aspirin's benefits are often not realised:

- It is an excellent pain-killer or analgesic.
- It is an effective anti-inflammatory medication.
- It quickly reduces fever.
- It is a safe medication if used correctly and in the appropriate dosage.

I use aspirin mainly for its pain-relieving and anti-inflammatory effectiveness. I immediately use it with patients suffering irritated tendons (tendonitis), irritated nerves (neuritis) or swollen joints.

After absorption, aspirin is rapidly distributed through all body tissues. It is excreted from the body mainly by the kidneys. About 50 per cent of a given dose is eliminated within 24 hours.

Rehabilitation should start as soon as the swelling stops. That means that within 48 hours after an injury, you should be working with a physiotherapist or trainer.

Rehabilitation should start as soon as the swelling stops.

CHAPTER 2

Physical activity and the growing skeleton

Physical activity, along with dietary and other lifestyle factors, is essential for the normal growth and development of the skeleton. As the body grows, the length of bones increases and with modelling and remodelling, modification of the bony architecture occurs.

During this period of growth, there are significant changes that occur in the composition of the bone, with increased mineralisation and associated stiffness and strength of the bones.

The growing skeleton appears more sensitive to loads produced by physical activity than its adult counterpart. The growing skeleton generally shows a positive response to endurance exercise of moderate intensity. Therefore it is important to appropriately monitor, control and supervise strenuous training programs involving young children. Intensive and repetitive exercise may have a deleterious effect on growing bones, with reductions in mineral apposition rates, strength and stiffness of bones. It is imperative to prescribe the right kind of exercise in the right amounts.

There are many specific injuries to children and young adolescents involving the growth aspects of the locomotor system. Any injury to a growth centre can be serious because growth centres are the mechanisms for growth of the long and flat bones of the body. Injuries to the growth centres can stunt growth or result in permanent joint deformity.

An injury can happen in many ways — a fall, a twist, a turn. The growth centre can be fractured — that is, broken, compressed or torn. Some or all of the growth cells may die and this can lead to altered patterns of growth development.

The injury may heal without any long-term deformity. Growth may be slowed temporarily until the fracture, or compression, of the growth centre has healed. Normal growth then continues. However, the growth centre can stop growing altogether if it has been significantly damaged.

The potential for deformity resulting from an injury to a growth centre is tremendous. Take, for example, an injury to the growth centre of the thigh bone — the femur. While the injured centre is healing, the other leg is growing, up to one to two centimetres a year. In the case of a 12-year-old boy, this could account for one leg being three or four centimetres shorter at the end of the growth period.

Sometimes, growth centres are only partially injured. This is an even more difficult medical situation because the growth centres will then usually cause only part of the bone to grow. In this case, if the child's bone grows out of line, it will be angular or crooked.

In the lower leg above the ankle, or in the lower arm above the wrist, there will be two bones growing. If only one is injured, then the growth discrepancy between the injured and and the non-injured bone must be looked at for its effect on the joint's function.

In a rapidly growing young adolescent, the injury to a knee from a side tackle is much more likely to be a growth centre fracture than a ligament injury.

A ligament injury would be more common in a fully grown person. In a young adolescent the essential thing to remember is that a ligament is stronger than a growth centre.

These growth centre injuries are usually seen under two circumstances. Sometimes the child is brought to a doctor with a routine fracture or a joint problem and the bones are X-rayed. When the bones are compared with the healthy bone or joint, there's an irregularity showing up on the X-ray in the growth centre. The other common way a child presents for treatment is when the parent notices a small limp or when a small bone is growing crookedly.

Injuries to growth centres and joints present very different problems for the young adolescent. There may be an injury to the joint surface cartilage and the maturing bone beneath the surface. This is called an 'intra-articular fracture' and is usually identified by careful X-ray examination of the joint. Invariably, such a fracture will require an operative procedure for proper re-establishment of a smooth joint surface.

At the time of early adolescence, children can commonly present with a unique growth plate injury known as a 'slipped epiphysis'. This is an injury to a growth centre. The most frequent is a slipped capital femoral epiphysis, that is, the ball of the hip joint becomes displaced.

This may happen gradually, or suddenly, during a sporting or physical event. The young adolescent is usually of a chubby body type and surgery may be required to prevent further slipping of the epiphysis. There's a 25 per cent chance of this happening to the other hip. So careful observation is important.

An 'avulsion fracture' is the name doctors give to fractures of the growth centres of flat bones. The most frequent sites of avulsions are

Any injury to a growth centre can be serious.

An 'avulsion fracture' is the name doctors give to fractures of the growth centres of flat bones.

Overuse syndromes happen when a child or a young adolescent exercises or trains too much.

Keep a sensible perspective on a child's physical limits.

the growth centres of the pelvic bone.

The large muscles of the back and abdomen extend into the top of the pelvis bone at the growth centre. Children and young adolescents who participate in sports that demand sudden twisting manoeuvres frequently sustain avulsion injuries.

Overuse Syndromes

Overuse syndromes in children and young adolescents are common. They happen when a child or a young adolescent exercises or trains too much. Frequently, the tissue cannot tolerate the strain and becomes injured. It's common to see young swimmers who train six hours a day, weightlifters who train twice a day six days a week and gymnasts who even live away from home with their coaches so they have more time to train! However, there's an upper limit to the amount of work that even a highly conditioned body can perform.

Never be carried away with enthusiasm. It's always wise to keep a commonsense perspective on a child's physical limits rather than expecting him/her to be able to achieve miracle performances.

Some individuals have a genetic predisposition to an overuse syndrome. In others, it may be hastened by lax ligaments or capsules supporting a joint.

Levels of injury

There are several levels, or grades, of overuse syndromes. In the mild grade, a child normally complains of a slight ache during exercise or sporting activities. Sometimes, the pain continues for a short time after the exercise ends. X-rays don't usually show any tissue changes.

In the next grade of overuse syndrome, the pain occurs during the performance, shortens participation time and continues after the performance has stopped. X-rays show early changes of bone and growth centres, particularly when compared with normal tissues.

In the third grade of overuse syndrome, the pain is significant during the performance as well as afterwards. It can last for many hours after the physical activity has ceased. The injury site swells and there's a difference in motion between the injured and the uninjured limb. X-ray changes are identifiable. This is usually in the form of excessive bone development or bone fragment development. At this particular level of overuse syndrome, it's important to understand that sporting activities have to be suspended for six to eight weeks and sometimes even longer. Sometimes, it's wise to apply a splint or cast to the limb or joint, to promote rest.

In the most severe form of overuse syndrome, the child is unable to perform for an extended period because of persistent pain in the injured area. After exercise, or stopping sporting activities, the pain lasts for more than 24 hours. X-rays show definite changes and usually the child or young adolescent has lost a full range of motion. In this final stage, the youngster has significant problems and it's best to advise rest for several months and, frequently, a change in sports.

PREVENTION OR RECOGNITION

It's important to listen to children and to encourage them to speak up when they're hurt. All too often, parents, coaches and team-mates encourage the injured youngster to play despite pain. This short-sighted attitude is almost guaranteed to lead to the development of level three and four overuse syndromes.

Pain is nature's way of telling your child that something is wrong. When it speaks, you should heed its advice! One of the classic examples of an overuse stress syndrome in children and young adolescents is the development of acute tendonitis in long-distance running.

The Australian Sports Medicine Federation, in conjunction with the American College of Sports Medicine, has laid down special guidelines to reduce overuse syndromes. (See page 34.) The guidelines particularly apply to long-distance running involving children and young adolescents. A child encouraged to participate at a higher rate than the recommended guidelines is at extreme risk of developing an overuse syndrome.

The best current treatments of overuse syndrome in children and young adolescents are prevention or early recognition. The tragedy is when a level three or four problem is diagnosed and the sad news has to be broken to the child and the parents. What a waste when it was all avoidable if caught early enough!

AVULSIONS

Avulsions involve much more than a muscle pull or strain. They are true fractures. The significance of diagnosing them correctly is that the healing time is significantly longer than with a muscle pull or strain.

An avulsion can take two to six months to heal. In general, it's not necessary to operate on an avulsion injury. The best treatment is:

- RICE
- rest and protection
- carefully increasing rehabilitation
- a cautious return to sporting activity.

OSTEOCHONDROSES

Osteochondroses are a group of disorders which occur in the growing areas of bone. They are simply a non-infectious interruption of the blood supply resulting in injured tissue in that area.

Pain is nature's way of telling your child that something is wrong.

Avulsions are true fractures.

The Growing Skeleton

Osteochondroses are non-infectious interruptions of the blood supply.

Causes

It usually begins with some single, or repetitive, injury (known as an 'episode trauma') to a bone or joint. This often occurs with overuse syndromes. Such situations affect the blood supply to the developing bone.

The symptoms usually follow excessive physical demands of sports participation and are most frequently identified during these early stages of growth development.

Any unusual compressive, or shearing, force may produce some change in the shape of the bone-cartilage unit or interfere with the area's blood supply. This changes its development and also its X-ray image.

Treatment

Early diagnosis of an osteochondrosis usually means healing without major deformity or disability. If it isn't easily identified, then it's possible that the symptoms will continue long-term with joint deformity and eventual impairment and disability.

Usually, doctors grade the severity of osteochondroses from grades one to four. Generally, the younger the child and the higher the grade, the more concern doctors have about the ultimate outcome.

There are two kinds of osteochondroses of childhood. Legg-Perthes syndrome is osteochondrosis of the femoral head, that is, the ball of the hip joint. Secondly, there's Kohler's syndrome — osteochondrosis of the navicular bone of the foot.

LEGG-PERTHES SYNDROME

Legg-Perthes syndrome usually occurs in children between four and eight years of age. The specific cause is unknown, but it's related to the restriction of blood supply to the head of the femur — the thigh bone — which becomes significantly altered with continued repetitive running and jumping. The child's complaint is usually one of the following:

- Pain about the hip and thigh.
- A painless limp.
- A mild limp with pain localising on the inner side of the knee.

The complaint of knee pain, when the problem is in the hip, occurs all too often in children. An important rule: when a child is complaining of knee pain, X-ray the hip.

Treatment

Non-surgical and surgical treatment are both used for Legg-Perthes syndrome. With an early diagnosis, non-surgical treatment with a brace will frequently produce satisfactory results. An operation may be necessary for a child with a long-standing history of, or advanced, deformity with progressive X-ray changes. Any child with a diagnosis of Legg-Perthes syndrome will probably be kept from participating in running and jumping sports for between 12 to 24 months.

A complaint of knee pain when the problem is really in the hip is common.

Kohler's syndrome

Kohler's syndrome is a similar process which occurs in the tarsal-navicular bone of the foot. The tarsal-navicular is in the inner part of the middle of the foot.

Treatment

The initial treatment is rest. The limitation of activities or the immobilisation of the foot in a splint or cast for six to eight weeks is usually sufficient to resolve the problem.

Osgood-Schlatter's syndrome

The most common form of osteochondrosis in early adolescence is Osgood-Schlatter's syndrome. It affects the front part of the upper tibia, just below the knee joint. This area can be felt as a bump, and is situated four to six centimetres below the kneecap.

When this cartilage converts to bone, or there's some repetitive stress on the attachment of the patella from the thigh muscles, a series of micro-fractures occur. These interrupt the normal blood supply and the normal conversion of the cartilage to bone, resulting in a tender bump. The major symptoms are localised pain and pain when pressure is applied to the bump.

The young athlete will typically complain of pain after activities such as running, jumping and kneeling.

Treatment

This is a condition which will heal when growth is completed. Until then, it's important to advise the young athlete to stay away from certain sporting activities that increase the pain. In some cases, it's necessary to apply a cast for six to eight weeks to aid the healing and prevent further irritation and disruption of the blood supply.

Scheuermann's disease

Other osteochondroses occur in the vertebral bodies of the spine during adolescence and account for postural deformities such as Scheuermann's disease.

Treatment

Once again, the key to success is early diagnosis, an appropriate change of activity, and prescribed exercises or the use of a cast or external bracing support.

The bone surfaces which form joints are covered with a glistening, white cartilage which is very slippery. Joint surface cartilage can be easily damaged. It can happen with a fall, a turn, a twist or a tackle. The cartilage, nourished and lubricated by joint fluid, has considerable elasticity and recovers from denting remarkably well.

Osteochondritis dissecans

Osteochondritis dissecans is a defect in the joint-bone cartilage of any synovial joint — the knee, wrist,

> *The key to success is early diagnosis.*

> *The cartilage has considerable elasticity and recovers from denting remarkably well.*

The Growing Skeleton

Joint surface cartilage can be easily damaged.

ankle or elbow. An X-ray of the area looks like a small excavation out of the joint surface. In time, the piece may loosen and cause pain. The 'dissecans' refers to a dissection of a loose piece from the surface of the joint.

In children, the dissecans usually remains seated in the divot — the excavated area. However, in athletes aged between 12 and 16, the divot sometimes falls free. When the piece does fall free into the joint, it is called a 'joint mouse' because it may wander around the joint.

In osteochondritis dissecans, the pain usually starts when the cartilage piece loosens from its bed. The movement of the piece causes the pain. If the child doesn't move the joint, no pain is created. Sometimes, a plain or regular X-ray of the joint doesn't identify the surface of the joint accurately enough.

In such cases, dye may have to be put into the joint to outline the joint surface, the fragment and the bone surface. This test is called an 'arthrogra'.

The status of a fragment can also be determined with an arthroscope, a joint telescope that can peer inside a narrow opening in the joint. This type of procedure is usually performed under general anaesthetic.

Treatment

In young children, the treatment for osteochondritis dissecans is rest. Sometimes, this means a splint or a cast. Rest works in 99 per cent of cases because the cartilage is still growing and usually covers the divot. There's usually no lasting deformity. Osteochondritis dissecans is usually a problem of diagnosis, not treatment.

In the 12- to 16-year-old age group, sometimes a splint or cast is recommended, but this would be better avoided if possible. If the fragment is present on a plain X-ray and the surface is intact, then the best way to proceed is to restrict sporting activities. Usually, this means three to six months of no sports. Sometimes a splint may be applied to the joint to restrict motion. But again, this is better avoided because the muscles around the joint will reduce in size and strength and this, in turn, slows rehabilitation and a return to physical activities.

I don't use cortisone injections, radiation or dietary changes. I have found they don't significantly help. Surgery must be considered if, after six months, the patient still experiences pain and the X-rays are unchanged, because in young people whose joints are still growing, it makes sense to try to stimulate the healing of the fragment. The operation stimulates the blood supply from the bone to the fragment.

If the athlete is skeletally mature and has completed bone growth, my experience is that it's almost biologically impossible for the cartilage to heal itself. Accordingly, an operation is the most effective solution.

In young children, the treatment for osteochondritis dissecans is rest.

DEVELOPMENTAL LESIONS

Without apparent reason, some children develop irregularities of bone during their growing process that result in minor developmental abnormalities. This growth irregularity occurs in approximately 20 per cent of the population.

There are two most common forms. Firstly, there are benign fibrocystic lesions, which grow near the growth centres. In the majority of children, these occur just above the knee joint. Secondly, there are osteochondromas, which are small projections of bone that extend away from the shaft of the bone. Sometimes they touch nerves or interfere with muscle function and cause pain.

Treatment

In most instances, these developmental lesions are identified on an X-ray taken because of some other problem. In most cases, they disappear or don't cause structural or physical interference. The best treatment is, therefore, instruction about the lesion. The child is usually permitted to continue with sporting activities.

In a rare instance, an osteochondroma will cause local discomfort or may interfere with a nerve or muscle function. In those cases, it may be necessary to surgically remove the abnormal bone growth.

TUMOURS

Other developmental lesions that may be of greater significance are tumours of the extremities. Not all tumours are malignant. However, even benign tumours can increase in size and may cause weakness and pain in the extremity.

Tumours and tumorous conditions of bone are most frequently brought to the attention of parents and physicians by a recent injury. In many cases, it's implied that the injury is the cause of the tumour or tumorous condition. In reality, the bone has been weakened by the underlying process, to the point where a small stress or trauma results in a mild fracture. This in turn causes the pain. When investigating the cause of the pain, X-rays reveal the abnormality of the bone consistent with some tumour or tumorous condition. In some cases, the tumour may be a benign lesion such as a bone cyst. The cyst has increased in size to a point where just throwing or kicking a ball creates enough stress to result in a fracture. Such fractures are known as 'pathological fractures'.

In other cases, the lesion may be caused by a bone tumour growing within the bone, or one that has spread to an area of bone from another site. Again, the bone is generally weakened to the extent that mild trauma results in a pathological fracture. This causes the pain and brings the child to the physician.

Without apparent reason, some children develop irregularities during their growing process.

Most developmental lesions are identified on an X-ray taken because of some other problem.

Don't diagnose problems as if they all are only sporting injuries.

LISTENING

Whenever a child complains of pain or appears to have sustained even an insignificant injury, you should listen! If questions remain, see the school trainer, nurse or doctor. Always remember that children and young adolescents who participate in sports are not immune to disease, tumours and other problems that afflict the general population. Parents, coaches and doctors should avoid the trap of diagnosing the problems which affect a young athlete solely in terms of injuries which can happen on the sporting field.

> **STOP**
>
> When a child complains of pain, **listen!**

CHAPTER 3

TRACK AND FIELD

Children are not little adults! That statement is never truer than when discussing running in athletics. The emphasis on running, particularly long-distance running, by children should never be on the duration or intensity of the activities. Rather, it should be on the pleasure of involvement as well as the development and appreciation of skills in throwing, running and jumping, all of which can be gained with the wide variety of excellent activities available in athletics.

The main sports injuries problems occur when there's overuse of various parts of the body due to excessive demands placed upon them. These excessive demands commonly include the intensity of the action performed, together with the duration of the stresses. This is particularly so in long-distance running.

Any problems with overuse injuries can be kept to a minimm provided these demands are monitored and controlled, particularly during the child's growth and development period.

PROBLEMATIC EXPECTATIONS

When there's a strong competitive element in such sports, problems arise more often with parents and coaches than with the children.

Without realising it, parents are often trying to fulfil their own desires and ambitions through their child's participation in competitive sports.

It's taking part and developing basic skills — rather than winning or losing — which are the most important things in the early formative period of a child's participation in physical activities.

Interestingly, when children are asked about their reasons for participating in physical activities, the competitive element is often not included in their top three or four priorities. Most important for children is the feeling of participation with their team-mates in physical activities which help them integrate within a particular social group. It is only when asked about the element of competition that many children reply that success in sport is important to them, to fulfill the expectations of their parents and their coaches.

As adults, we should be more aware of our children's desires and expectations, and respond to them when developing and organising their physical activities. The goals should be participation by our children in many and varied physical activities. Athletics can be an excellent vehicle for this, provided the emphasis is on the child's growth and development, with an ever-increasing acquisition of desired skills, rather than on the ambitious pursuit of medals and the victory dais at all costs. Success will come naturally when the child has physically and emotionally matured.

> *Schedule sporting activities in ways that reduce the risk of serious injuries.*

Good Organisation

If you have ever been to an athletics competition, you can understand what an organisational nightmare it can be, with so many small children in such an enclosed area performing such a variety of physical activities simultaneously! It's therefore imperative that the organisation is of a high standard, because accidents can easily happen in such situations.

Hazards

The organising committee needs tight coordination so that they schedule sporting activities in ways that reduce the risk of serious injuries — making sure that the track events don't involve children running across the path of field events competitors, for example.

The actual arena, including the track, should always be checked for areas of damage which could cause runners to twist their ankles or fall over and sustain cuts or bruises. The arena's inner surface should also be checked for protruding objects, such as sprinkler systems or other pieces of equipment thoughtlessly left lying about. These can cause serious injury to participants concentrating more on their activities than on what may be under their feet.

With such events as the long jump and the triple jump, the run-up should also be checked for damage. Most importantly, the landing pit should be thoroughly inspected — make sure the sand is raked and there are no hidden objects concealed in the landing area.

Wet weather

It's very important that the sand is dry. If it's been extremely wet before the competition, and almost muddy in the landing area, then the staging of that particular event should be cancelled. Serious injuries can occur to the knees and hips of competitors landing in a very wet, sloppy pit area.

I had an example of such an incident when working in Toronto, Canada. I was at the Sports Clinic with Dr Robert Jackson when a young boy arrived with a badly swollen knee. He related how he had been long jumping the previous day when he had landed and slipped in the wet pit and felt his knee hyperextend — that is, go beyond full straightening. He was certain something major had snapped. An extensive examination showed he had damaged his posterior cruciate ligament — one of the ligaments in the middle of the knee at the back. He had, in fact, sustained a complete rupture of the posterior cruciate ligament as well as damage to the menisci — the cartilages — on both sides of the knee. After performing an arthroscopy, his knee was placed in a plaster cast to heal over six to eight weeks.

As we left the operating room, Dr Jackson was still perplexed about

> *The arena should always be checked for areas of damage which could cause runners to twist their ankles or fall.*

how such a serious injury could occur. The answer wasn't long in coming.

We were reading a newspaper in the surgeons' room while waiting for the next patient to come from the ward. There, on the back page, was a photograph of this boy long jumping in the pouring rain and landing in this pit that was awash with water and sloppy sand. The photograph was a classic illustration of his leg hyperextending as his foot hit and slipped forward approximately two feet without any grip in the sand. It was immediately clear how this serious injury had happened.

I must therefore re-emphasise the importance of an awareness of climatic conditions when staging events, particularly athletics. Serious injuries can be avoided by deferring certain events if the climatic conditions demand it — if there is water on the track or in the landing pit.

High jump hazards

Landing pit hazards are also overlooked with dire results every year for high jumpers. Such pits are usually constructed with large rubber pontoons placed together to provide a softly cushioned landing when performing the high jump, or with older athletes, the pole vault. It's very important to have a marshal or organiser keeping a close eye on the rubber pontoons or mattresses.

There are many examples of serious injuries being caused by inadequate divisioning of the rubber pontoons, resulting in an unnecessarily heavy landing. The most important thing to do is make sure that the rubber pontoons don't separate in the middle — particularly in the area where the athletes usually land.

I have experienced several cases where a young athlete has successfully cleared the bar only to disappear between the pontoons, with only his feet visible!

As luck would have it, there were no serious injuries but it's inevitable that unless such risks are minimised with more care and thoughtfulness, serious injuries will occur to the back or legs. Talented young athletes are too valuable to subject to such unnecessary risks.

Hot weather

The other climatic condition to be wary of is extremely hot or humid weather, especially when you are attempting to stage middle- to long-distance running events. Use of head gear and sunscreens is extremely important in very hot and sunny weather.

> *Make sure your rubber pontoons or mattresses are in good condition and placed correctly.*

> *The sand must be dry.*

STOP
Postpone events if the weather is too hot or too wet.

> *The emphasis should be on the pleasure of involvement.*

> *The goal should be participation in many and varied activities.*

LONG-DISTANCE RUNNING

Extensive experience in staging long-distance running events for children has led to many important guidelines being established by the Australian Sports Medicine Federation and the American College of Sports Medicine. All of these are based on the underlying truth that children are not little adults. Certain stresses in long-distance running, which adults may be able to handle, may be beyond children. I believe that children under the age of 12 shouldn't run in long-distance events beyond 5 to 10 kilometres.

In my opinion, the staging of marathons for young children is fraught with danger. This becomes even more critical when staging long-distance running events in warmer, humid weather.

For events involving children running 5 kilometres or more, organisers must be aware of the temperature and humidity. If the temperature is beyond 27°C, serious consideration should be given to postponing the event.

DEHYDRATION

It's important to understand that children have a significantly different ratio of body surface area to body mass from adults. This means that children have a larger surface area through which to lose water and salt, in the form of perspiration, and do so at a greater rate than adults. Simply put, kids cook quicker! This is the body's way of attempting to cool its core temperature, which rises in hot weather, particularly when performing a strenuous physical act such as running. Thus, a young child can dehydrate at a greater rate than an adult in the same climatic conditions, when performing proportionately the same physical activities.

AVOID FATALITIES

It's therefore vital that rehydration stations, providing water and drinks for participants, be placed at every ½ to 1 kilometre along the route of an event of 5 kilometres or more. An equally important requirement is that first aid stations, staffed by qualified personnel with training in the management of dehydration and other running problems, be placed at every 2 kilometres.

By following these clear and simple guidelines when staging a running event for young children, potentially fatal situations can be easily avoided. The emphasis for young children participating in physical activity should be on fun, growth and development. It is certainly not an opportunity for parents to place their children in stressful situations in an atmosphere of intense competitiveness.

> **STOP**
> The emphasis should be on fun, growth and development.

THE RIGHT SHOES

Injury prevention measures in distance running should start with running shoes. A good pair doesn't necessarily mean an expensive pair.

The following are important guidelines to consider when selecting a new pair of running shoes or considering whether to replace an old pair.

1 Shoes should be well fitting — not too tight and not too loose.

2 Shoes should have some flexibility in the mid-sole. Test this by bending the shoe back towards the heel with your hand. You should be able to do this, without excessive force, to about 50° from the horizontal. The mid-sole of the shoe should be firm while at the same time allowing enough flexibility for variation of movement during the running phases.

3 Shoes should be appropriate for foot shape. Observe the shape of your child's feet, because most feet curve slightly inwards towards the toe. Just to make life interesting, sometimes a foot may be absolutely straight. There are shoes which are made straight and lasted so that the sole is in a straight line. Alternatively, there are shoes which bend slightly towards the inside, particularly in that part of the shoe towards the toe box.

4 Different styles suit different runners. If you remove the insole from the shoe, you will see that some shoes are made in a style which is called 'split-lasted' in which the shoe's last is split and then sewn together. Other shoes are 'board-lasted'. This type of stiffer shoe should be used by heavier runners, while split-lasted shoes are better suited to lighter runners.

5 Shoes should have adequate room in the toe box for all the toes to fit without cramping. Otherwise, blisters can form, particularly on the inner side of the big toe and the outer side of the little toe.

6 Probably the most important consideration in the analysis of running shoes is the heel-counter. This is the cuff of the heel at the back of the shoe. It should be deep enough to allow support of the entire heel portion of the foot. You should check that it's firm enough to provide good support for the heel through the various phases of running. Most good running shoes have a heel-counter made of a polyurethane material. But there are some shoes which still use cardboard. The way to tell is that the shoes with cardboard are softer when you push your thumb into this part of the shoe. These shoes should be avoided. Cardboard weakens when it gets wet and the support of the heel counter reduces dramatically. This in turn significantly affects the support of the foot during running.

7 It's very important that there's not excessive wearing of the insole, the outer sole or the shoe in the region of the heel. This can cause a twisting effect on the heel which can lead to injuries of the ankle joint and the joint just below this. These are important joints in maintaining stability of the foot in twisting and turning manoeuvres. So check the sole in the heel portion of the shoe very carefully.

8 Make sure that there are adequate groovings in the tread of the outer sole to enable a good grip on a loose surface or in wet, slushy conditions such as prevail when running on grass.

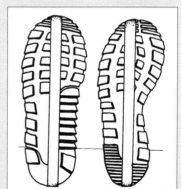

A straight-lasted shoe (left) and a curve-lasted shoe (right).

Children are not little adults!

Children under the age of 12 shouldn't run in events longer than 5 to 10 kilometres.

Guidelines for Children in Running

Recommendations from the Australian Sports Medicine Federation and the American College of Sports Medicine, endorsed by the American Academy of Pediatrics.

1 All children should have a musculo-skeletal assessment before embarking upon a training/competition program of long-distance running.
2 Running events primarily designed for adults are not recommended for children before physical maturation. Under no circumstances should a full marathon be attempted by children or adolescents.
3 The maximum training distance should be three times the competition distance. Children known to be physically immature for their age should be limited to the maximum recommended distance for the age group below their own.
4 Regular long periods of running on hard surfaces should be avoided.
5 Children should not be encouraged to participate in competitions designed for adults.
6 Weather conditions should be cool.
7 Children should be taught about ingestion of fluids before and during a race or training session.
8 Appropriate clothing should be worn.
9 There is a danger that the time required for training/competition in distance running may preclude a child from enjoying a wide range of social experiences. Study, mixing with other children and developing other skills are important in normal growth and development.
10 Recommended maximum competitive distances:

Age	Distance
Under 12 years	5 kilometres
13–15 years	10 kilometres
15–16 years	½ Marathon (21 kilometres)
16–18 years	30 kilometres
18 and over	Marathon (42 kilometres)

Muscle Injuries

The most common injuries in athletic events, particularly running, are those to muscles and tendons as well as to some joints involving the ligaments and capsules.

In short running events such as sprints or middle-distance running, or in jumping and throwing events, one incident of overstress can damage a muscle or tendon. Typically, the muscle or tendon is suddenly stressed beyond its capabilities at one particular instant. This causes some damage to muscle fibres whether they be in the middle portion of the muscle or where the muscle becomes a tendon at the attachment to a bone.

A muscle usually begins at a bone. It then develops into a muscle belly made up of many thousands of muscle fibres. This then tapers down into a muscle tendon junction continuing on as a tendon. It then inserts itself onto another bone, acting across a joint to enable the movement of part of a limb. This is, in turn, acted upon by this muscle-tendon unit.

The various areas where damage can occur from an overstress situation are at the origin of the muscle, within the muscle belly itself, at the junction of the muscle and tendon and either within the tendon substance or near its insertion on the bone.

At each of these areas, when overstress occurs, there's damage to the muscle and/or tendon fibres. The athlete immediately experiences pain which can prevent the completion of the activity.

In sprinters and jumpers, this muscle injury commonly occurs in

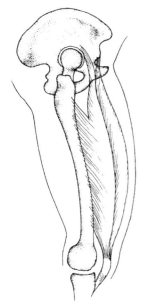

One of the thigh muscles commonly injured from an overstress.

the hamstrings and thigh muscles. But it occasionally strikes in the calf muscle extending into the Achilles tendon. In middle-distance runners, the injuries mainly involve the legs and again can occur in the hamstring muscles, the calf muscles and the Achilles tendon.

For those who participate in throwing sports, injuries can occur in the legs, and there is also the possibility of muscle and/or tendon damage in the upper arms. Particularly at risk are the biceps and triceps muscles and also the muscles supporting the shoulder joint.

Treatment

Immediately a young athlete experiences pain in one of these areas, stop the activity and apply ice, in the form of an ice pack wrapped in a wet towel over the painful area. Apply the ice pack firmly with an elasticised bandage for compression.

If possible, elevate the injured area to help reduce fluid formation, whether it be damage to muscles or tendons.

Usually, the muscle or tendon damage in young children and adolescents is only mild or moderately severe. You will significantly reduce pain and irritation to the damaged area by applying RICE (rest, ice, compression and elevation) over the next 24 to 48 hours. Following this treatment, simple stretching manoeuvres can be started. These will enable the muscles to resume some of

Provide water and drinks every half to one kilometre along the route of any event that is 5 kilometres or more in distance.

One incident of overstress can damage a muscle or tendon.

Simple stretching manoeuvres speed rehabilitation.

their normal activities without allowing excessive contraction of the muscle or the scar tissue. This speeds rehabilitation and also prevents excessive stiffness and contracture.

If the area of tissue damage is localised, ice massage can be performed for three or four days while doing these stretching manoeuvres. Hold the ice in a towel. Alternatively, use ice which has been frozen in a polystyrene cup with the lip of the cup broken away to expose the ice. You can then apply the ice directly applied to the skin, massaging in the direction of the muscle fibres to relieve muscle spasm and tightness. This is particularly effective following an exercise program which has considerably stretched the muscle.

There are specific exercises to initially stretch the muscle after injury. The exercises vary depending upon the area of the body where the injury has occurred, the nature of the accident and the muscle which has been damaged.

These exercises should be done

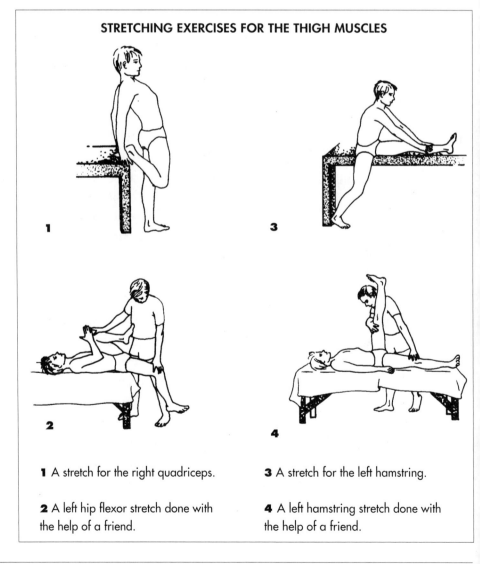

STRETCHING EXERCISES FOR THE THIGH MUSCLES

1 A stretch for the right quadriceps.

2 A left hip flexor stretch done with the help of a friend.

3 A stretch for the left hamstring.

4 A left hamstring stretch done with the help of a friend.

without resistance or any weights, and gradually, within the limits of pain, the injured person should increase the intensity and number of repetitions to stretch and strengthen the muscle-tendon structures.

Once the young athlete can fully stretch the affected muscle-tendon unit without pain, and has also undergone at least two or three days of intense strengthening exercises, then some training can be resumed. This should specifically involve the previously damaged muscle-tendon unit.

It's very important that the young athlete undergoes a specific retraining program which includes education about how the injury happened. This promotes an understanding of how to avoid reinjury.

Emphasis should be on an adequate warm-up before training or competition, which involves not only specific stretching exercises for the previously damaged muscle-tendon unit, but also exercises that stretch the commonly used muscle groups for that particular physical activity.

After training or a competition, it may also be advisable to apply ice for about 10 to 15 minutes to the previously injured muscle. This is particularly useful in the first two to three weeks after return to normal training and competition, to prevent any further accumulation of fluid in the injured area. This practice also prevents any spasm or contraction of the muscle-tendon unit.

Preventive measures such as a proper warm-up, a stretching program and icing down after intensive physical activities following an injury, help prevent recurrence of the injury. They also make the athlete aware of how tissues can be injured and the best ways to avoid such injuries in the future.

ILIOTIBIAL BAND

Running injuries predominantly involve the legs and, in children, the feet, the Achilles tendon and a band of tissue that runs down the outer side of the thigh from the hip towards the outer surface of the knees.

This band of tissue is known as the iliotibial band. It comprises a tendinous substance that helps the knee maintain full extension or straightening. It has an auxiliary significance at the hip joint, particularly in running up or down hills.

This band can become irritated in three common places. The first is near the hip bone. You can feel it on the outer surface of the buttocks at the commencement of the thigh. Here, the band of tissue can rub across the bony prominence at the upper part of the thigh bone. It's here that a bursa, or sac, that helps in the gliding of this band across this bone can become inflamed. A bursitis can form where excess fluid collects in the sac. The area becomes quite tender when touched or after running some distance.

The band itself can also become

A specific retraining program is very important.

Always start with an adequate warm-up.

> *Apply ice after training or competition.*

irritated in this region. It becomes tender to touch and also tends to become sore soon after the start of running, particularly when trying to run up or down hills.

The second area where this band of tissue can become inflamed is in the mid-portion of the tissue. This isn't as common as in the upper aspect of the thigh. Nor is it as common as in the lower aspect, where the band runs across the outer aspect of the knee towards its attachment on the tibia — the large bone in the lower leg below the knee.

The region of the iliotibial band at the knee joint can become irritated when friction occurs as the band moves slightly across the knee joint when the joint moves from full straightening to full bending. As the band of tissue glides across the bone, it can become irritated and inflamed. This causes pain and irritation when attempting to run and, sometimes, when trying to jump.

> *Once the inflammation and the pain have subsided, gentle stretching can be performed.*

ILIOTIBIAL BAND EXERCISE

Stand with one leg behind the other leg. Bend with arms outstretched to touch the inner side of the heel of the foot that is behind the front leg. Hold stretch for 5 to 10 seconds and repeat ten times. Then cross the legs in the opposite direction and repeat the stretch, bending to again touch the inner heel of the foot that is behind the leg in front.

Treatment

The best treatment for this condition is to avoid the activity that caused the irritation for a while. If a specific correlation between the injury and running on hills is found, this should also be avoided for four to six weeks.

Ice massage is also very beneficial for this condition, using the method previously described — an ice block held in a towel or a refrigerated polystyrene cup of ice. Where the specific irritation is localised, a rhythmical ice massage is good for reducing inflammation.

If the inflammation persists, seek medical advice. A mild oral anti-inflammatory medication is often prescribed to help with the ice massage in reducing the inflammation and scarring in the area of tissue damage.

Once the inflammation and the pain have subsided, gentle stretching can be performed. There are specific exercises for the iliotibial band. They should be performed in groups of three repetitions followed by the application of ice massage.

Jogging can recommence once the athlete is able to fully stretch the iliotibial band without pain and when there's no specific pain at rest. There can be a gradual increase (over a two- to three-week period) in the running intensity, duration and frequency. But it's best to avoid hill running until the athlete can run without pain for a considerable length of time on flat terrain.

A SAFE RETURN WITHOUT REINJURY?

There are four main aspects in any running program:
- The number of runs each week.
- The distance or duration of each run.
- The intensity of the session, that is, the speed of the run and whether sprinting or other activities are incorporated.
- The nature of the terrain, particularly the variation between flat and hilly surfaces.

Reintroducing a running program after an injury should involve gradually increasing each of these variables, one at a time. This allows the body to readjust without risking a recurrence of an injury or the development of a different one.

I usually recommend that the runner return to jogging, possibly two to three times a week, over an extended period, which may be six to eight weeks. Keep the distance to maybe a third of the distance of the usual training program. Then gradually increase the duration of the run, still running two or three times a week.

Once you have reached normal training distance, gradually increase the number of runs to the number performed before the injury. Then introduce changes to the intensity of the runs. Finally, introduce variations to the terrain, particularly taking note of the type of injury sustained earlier. For example, if a child is recovering from an iliotibial band injury, you should reintroduce the child to hill running very slowly, as the last variable in the resumption of the training program.

With the popularity of long-distance running there's been an upsurge in the development of stress fractures.

INFLAMMATION OF THE PATELLA TENDON

Another common running injury in young runners is inflammation of the patella tendon.

This is a tendon extending from the thigh muscle to surround the kneecap (the patella) continuing on to insert in the front of the tibia (lower leg bone below the knee joint).

Inflammation of this tendon in runners can occur just above or below the kneecap and also at the point of insertion on the tibia.

Treatment
Again, the cornerstone of treatment is rest and the avoidance of running until the inflammation has subsided. Ice massage should also be applied, together with specific stretching exercises for the quadriceps/hamstrings.

STRESS FRACTURES

Fortunately, stress fractures are not as common in young children and adolescents as they are in adult long-distance runners. But with the popularity of long-distance running and the dramatic distances that young children have been running over the last few years, there's been an upsurge in the development of stress fractures in the bones of the lower limbs — particularly the tibia and the fibula (the two bones of the lower leg) and

Prolonged overuse can cause stress fractures.

> ### DIAGNOSING A STRESS FRACTURE IS DIFFICULT
>
> Sometimes it can be very difficult to make an accurate diagnosis of a stress fracture from an X-ray. The only clinical finding is often an area of diffuse pain in the lower leg.
>
> A specific investigation known as a bone scan is often required. This involves a radioactive dye being injected into the vein. Over a period of several hours, the dye circulates through the body and concentrates in areas of calcium deposits or new bone formation.
>
> Where there's a fracture, calcium deposits increase as part of the overall bone healing process. There's an increase in the uptake of dye in such an area, which shows up as a 'hot spot' on the scan, clearly identifying the position of the stress fracture.

also some small bones of the foot.

Stress fractures are usually caused by prolonged overuse. But on occasions they can be caused by one specific instance of overstress which results in damage to the structure of the bone.

In the young runner, irritation of the Achilles tendon is quite common.

Treatment

Treatment of stress fractures is usually the same as for a normal fracture of the bone — except that, on occasions, the application of a plaster of Paris cast is not required as there's no deformity.

Provided the young athlete avoids excessive stress on that injured part of the body, the main treatment is rest, to allow the bone to heal. This usually takes four to six weeks.

ACHILLES TENDON PROBLEMS

In the young runner, irritation of the Achilles tendon is quite common. Inflammation can result in the lower part of the calf extending to behind the ankle and even down to the insertion of the tendo-Achilles on the back of the heel bone.

Usually, inflammation of the Achilles tendon occurs as the result of an overuse syndrome. Excessive use of the calf muscle is often the cause.

Treatment

The treatment should therefore involve rest, ice massage and specific stretching and strengthening exercises for the calf muscle, as shown in the diagrams on page 41.

These exercises should be done regularly: two or three times a day, with three sets of 20 repetitions of each exercise. It's also very important to strengthen the calf muscles before returning to a running program.

With any muscle or tendon injury, that combination of stretching and strengthening exercises must be performed in the rehabilitation period. Lack of strength in the muscle

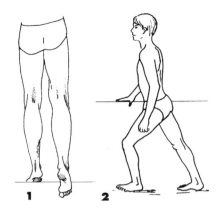

CALF STRETCHING AND STRETCHENING EXERCISES

1 Toe raises for calf muscle strengthening help prevent Achilles tendon injuries.
2 Combined calf stretching and Achilles tendon exercise. To complete the exercise reverse the leg position and stretch again.

is a common causes of reinjury to the area when an athlete returns to a strenuous activity such as running.

COMMON FOOT INJURIES IN LONG-DISTANCE RUNNING

Finally, I would like to discuss briefly some injuries which can occur in the foot as a result of long-distance running.

INFLAMMATION

The most common is inflammation to the band of tissue which runs across the sole of the foot from the front of the heel bone to the bases of all of the toes. Known as the plantar fascia, it's a very important ligament which helps maintain the arches of the foot and prevents the forebones of the foot spreading out, particularly when taking weight on the foot.

This band of tissue or ligament can become inflamed near its attachment on the front of the heel bone, commonly on the inner side of the foot. But the inflammation can also occur in the mid-substance of the ligament, usually on the inner surface. On occasions, it can extend to the bases of the toes. This is a common and quite painful running

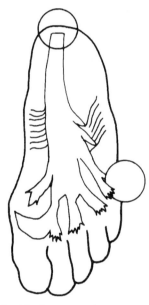

Plantar fascitis. It commonly occurs at the point of attachment to the heel or near its insertion at the base of the toes. Inflammation can occur on the sole of the foot involving the large supporting ligament.

injury. If the young athlete tries to keep running or engage in other strenuous activities, severe pain can result. Even walking becomes painful.

> *Blisters should be treated promptly and carefully.*

Treatment

No attempt should be made to run. Apply ice massage and possibly use oral anti-inflammatory medication. If the pain due to inflammation persists, physiotherapy (in the form of ultrasonic treatment) may be necessary.

If massage doesn't resolve the problem and the inflammation is quite localised, then an injection of cortisone steroid and a long-lasting local anaesthetic may be necessary to specifically reduce the inflammation in this area. Once this has been administered, it's essential that the athlete completely rest the area for one or two days. This may require the use of crutches, with a gradual increase of weight bearing over seven to ten days.

BLISTERS

Other common foot injuries in runners include the formation of blisters, most frequently over the toes, particularly the inner surface of the big toe and in the outer aspect of the little toe, and also at the back of the heel. This can be caused by an excessive amount of running or by ill-fitting shoes.

Treatment

Blisters should be treated promptly and carefully. Otherwise, infections can cause significant problems in the feet. Not only will they prevent the athlete returning to running, but they can also cause much more generalised problems if the infection becomes severe and involves lymph glands.

Usually it's best to let the blister burst, or puncture it with a hot needle which has been sterilised in boiling water. Allow the skin overlying the blister to remain, unless it's torn away. It's preferable not to cut this skin away because it provides a protective layer over the underlying raw area of new skin.

HELPFUL HINTS

- Always have a well-organised program. Remember that children in an enclosed area, such as a track and field arena, can be seriously injured if events are not well supervised and not thoughtfully placed so as to minimise the risk of injuries.

- Always clear the track of any dangerous objects, particularly in running events, because young athletes concentrating intensely on their activities can easily miss any objects lying on the track or in the centre arena.

- Make sure that the landing pits for the long jump, triple jump and high jump are adequate. and appropriately maintained and supervised by an adult. Be alert to the serious injuries which can occur to the spine, pelvis and points of the lower limbs due to inadequate landing pits or inappropriately-placed rubber pontoons in the high jump area.

- Shoes are the most important equipment for young athletes engaging in running. Always make sure that:

They are well fitting and have a firm and well-positioned heel counter.

The mid-sole isn't too rigid or too flexible.

The outer sole has a good tread and isn't excessively flared in the region of the heel.

The toe box is of an adequate size to prevent excessive rubbing of the toes, which could cause blisters.

- With running, an adequate warm-up is a must and should include special stretching exercises for muscles in the lower limbs, such as the calf, thigh and hamstrings.

- Common injuries in athletics are to muscles and tendons, caused by one overstress incident, particularly in sprinting, jumping or throwing. This usually involves the muscles and tendons of the lower limbs. Treatment should include rest, ice massage, and avoiding the activities which caused the problems.

- Once the pain caused by any inflammation has subsided, immediately begin specific strengthening and stretching exercises. These should involve not only the muscle and tendon unit, but also other associated muscles in the specific area of the injured part of the body.

- Children and young adolescents are not little adults. They cannot be expected to perform the same activities at the same intensity as adults. Thus, excessive long-distance running is fraught with danger and can cause serious problems which affect the growth and development of the child.

CHAPTER 4

Football: Australian Rules, Rugby League, Rugby Union and Soccer

Injury Prevention

Before discussing the most common injuries, let's focus attention on prevention — the most important aspect of all for football or any other type of sport. Areas to consider include: the playing area; equipment; training; referees and umpires.

The playing area

The Australian climate is so good, even in winter, that most football games are played outdoors, except for the recent development of indoor soccer. It's essential that someone carefully check the playing surface before the game starts.

You should look for any protruding objects on the ground which could cause serious injury if a player fell on them. Don't forget underground sprinkler systems which may not be adequately covered. The ground surface should be evenly grassed. Although this is clearly difficult in the summer months, remember that large areas of clay or dirt without an even cover of grass can cause serious abrasions and damage when players fall or twist onto such a surface at high speed.

It's also very important that the boundary line be well away from any fence or other fixed object close to the ground. I believe that about 2 metres (at least 6 feet) should be allowed between a boundary and any fence so that players can avoid serious injury if they run into the fence or are pushed out of the field by an opposing player.

Goal posts should be well padded. Many young players have been seriously injured when running into such uprights at high speed. The risk of serious injuries can easily be minimised, if not eliminated altogether.

Protective equipment

In the codes of football played in Australia, there's very little protective equipment used, except for shoulder pads by rugby players. These should be checked regularly to make sure they are in good order and that they are the right size for the player's age and build. More harm can occur when a player is wearing protective equipment which is too large or too small.

Padded knee bandages are helpful for young players troubled by soreness on the front of their knees. This particularly happens in the early part of the season when the weather is warm and the ground is hard. The wearing of such knee and elbow braces can help prevent any further damage to the knee or elbow joints.

Check those boots

Boots are probably the most important item of equipment of all for football players. They should be a good-fitting pair, checked regularly to make sure they are not too small or too large. The stops, or studs, should be an appropriate size. Certainly don't have any sharp or protruding nails or sharp pieces of nylon which can inflict considerable damage to the skin and soft tissues if applied vigorously to an opponent either intentionally or by accident.

A major problem with boots, particularly with young footballers, is that the boots marketed in Australia are low-cut types which don't provide enough ankle support. These are the boots worn by professional footballers and are therefore easily marketed by the major companies to aspiring younger players.

Unbeknown to the majority of young footballers, the professional footballers have their ankles strapped with non-elastic tape which is quite rigid. This precaution is taken when training as well as when playing. Although professional footballers prefer low-cut boots for mobility and speed, the added protection of strapping helps minimise twisting injuries which can occur to the ankle joint.

As young footballers don't have the luxury of such protection, I strongly advise that footballers under the age of 16 should be encouraged to wear higher-cut boots to avoid injury.

There's much hard evidence that high-cut boots don't impede mobility or speed of movement. But they certainly give the player added protection from the frequent twisting and turning of the ankle and foot in all codes of football.

The real problem parents have is that the boots are not readily available. They also have to convince their young budding champions that low-cut boots won't somehow transform them into superstars.

Pre-season training

It's very important for players participating in a contact sport to reach and maintain a minimum fitness level before the season begins. This enables

More harm can occur when a player is wearing protective equipment which is too large or too small.

Boots should be checked regularly.

Good pre-season training produces strong, flexible muscles.

individual players to attain a skill level necessary for their particular code of football. Players can then perform in a game, better able to withstand the gruelling stresses applied to the body.

Thorough pre-season preparation produces muscles which are flexible and strong, as well as supporting joints which are aware of what is required of them for a particular movement. They are better able to withstand the intensity of forces and stresses applied to them during decisive moments of the game.

Know the rules

Don't just think you know the rules, make certain you do. Significantly fewer injuries occur when all players know and apply the rules of a particular code.

The ground surface should be evenly grassed.

Other preventive factors are the umpires and officials. It's imperative they know and understand the rules and apply them consistently.

Less ignorance by all involved avoids unnecessary confusion and conflict between players, with fewer injuries likely. Injuries, however, can only be reduced, never eliminated. The very nature of football and other vigorous contact sports inevitably means players being injured.

Muscle Injuries

In all codes of football and contact sports, direct force applied to the body can result in bruising to the soft tissues beneath the skin and, more importantly, to the muscles which lie just deep enough in the soft tissues.

This direct force results in damage to the muscle tissue. This is known as a 'haematoma' — a bleeding within the muscle due to damage of the muscle fibres and the small blood vessels within the tissues.

Clearly, in soccer, these injuries usually occur to the legs from the hips down. But in rugby codes and Australian Rules football, direct injuries can occur to any part of the body, particularly the shoulders and the upper arms as well as the thighs and the hips. The extent of the injury is directly related to the amount of damaged muscle tissue.

A muscle strain is also damage to the muscle tissue and results in bleeding and swelling. However, this

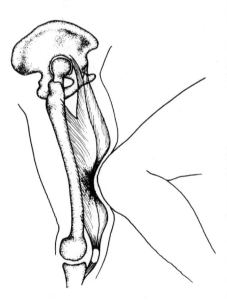

Damage to the thigh muscle usually occurs from a direct blow by an opponent. The damaged muscle usually bleeds, forming a haematoma.

happens not because of an external force, but rather from the tearing of the muscle fibres when excessive internal forces are applied to the muscle.

Either way, the effect of damage to the muscle tissue is the same. Therefore, the same treatment is used for both a muscle contusion caused by an external force and a muscle strain due to an internal force.

Treatment

Before describing how to treat a muscle tissue injury, I would like to give you an example of how not to treat such an injury. I hope this will reinforce the advice for appropriate treatment.

Again, when I was the club doctor at Prahran Football Club, I was attending training on a Tuesday night when a father came in, concerned about how slowly a wound his son had sustained the previous Saturday was healing.

He then brought in the 14-year-old boy who walked with a noticeable limp. He described how his left thigh had been hit by an opponent's knee and that the leg had quickly become swollen. The local trainer had told him to go home that night and have a hot bath. The next day, he was advised to run some laps of the oval in an attempt to stretch the muscle and 'run out' the injury. This was before the development of the Australian Sports Trainers Association.

I then asked the young boy to

STRENGTHENING EXERCISES FOR THE THIGH MUSCLES

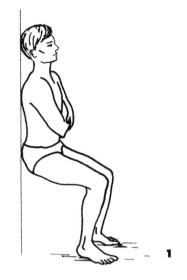

1 In the sitting position, hold the body against a wall.

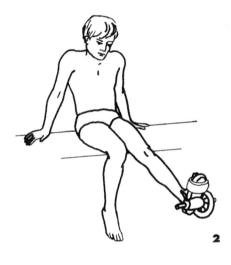

2 This is an isotonic exercise for the quadriceps using a foot weight. Bend the knee at 90° and then lift until straight.

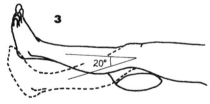

3 Another isotonic quadriceps exercise. The knee joint is moved through about 20°. This exercise is used after a recent injury or knee surgery.

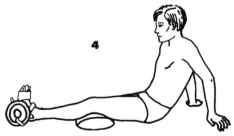

4 A foot weight can be used for a more limited isotonic quadriceps exercise.

Goal posts should be well padded.

Padded knee bandages are helpful.

remove his trousers. It was no surprise to see an extremely swollen left thigh. It was about 8 cm larger in circumference than the right thigh and was extremely tender to touch.

I estimate that he had bled 2 to 3 litres of blood into that left thigh. In fact, the fluid was now moving down into the region of his left knee and also down into the left calf muscle. Without the right treatment, there would have been further bleeding into the thigh and possibly calcification of the haematoma which is known as 'myositis ossificans'. Unfortunately, this young boy had been given the wrong advice and had applied all the wrong principles of treating a muscle or soft tissue injury.

RICE

The cornerstone of treatment for soft tissue bruising, muscle bruising or tearing is RICE:

- REST
- ICE
- COMPRESSION
- ELEVATION

With the simple application of these four basic principles, you can avoid serious complications which could result in permanent damage. (The RICE treatment is explained on pages 16 and 17.)

Once the pain and swelling have subsided, gentle exercise can start, within the limitations of pain. That is, if it's too painful to stretch the muscle any further, then restrict the exercises to the range of movement that can be tolerated. Increase the exercises gradually until a full range of movement is possible. Only then can the player resume more strenuous activities like running, twisting, stretching and eventually participation in the full training program.

JOINT INJURIES

Joint injuries are quite common in all three codes of football. In soccer, they usually involve the ankle and knee joints as well as hand injuries from contact with the ball. In rugby codes and Australian Rules football, joint injury commonly involves the hands and the shoulder girdle, the knee and the ankle joints.

FINGER DISLOCATIONS

With hand injuries, full or partial dislocations of the small joints of the fingers are quite common.

Treatment

No matter how urgent the demands of the game, dislocation of the small joint in the finger should mean immediate splinting. It's a simple matter to strap the affected finger to one either side of it. This provides an excellent splint.

The player should then be sent for an X-ray to make sure there isn't any significant damage to the joint or to the adjacent bone. Usually, there won't be any significant joint or bone damage. With the application of ice and appropriate splinting, the swelling reduces and movement resumes over the next two to three days. The player is then able to return to competition without any significant disruption.

However, I always advise that a player continue strapping the injured finger to the accompanying one. This allows full movement in the affected joint. Also, the strapping should be done at every training session and during competition for the next two to three weeks.

SHOULDER GIRDLE INJURIES

All injuries to the shoulder girdle are potentially serious. In rugby codes and Australian Rules football, injuries to the shoulder girdle usually occur in the form of a dislocation to the shoulder joint.

This often happens when the arm is forced backwards when tackling a player or when landing awkwardly.

Treatment

If the player appears distressed and holds the arm in a protective manner against the side of the body, it's possible they have injured the shoulder girdle. Carefully observe the shoulder girdle to see if it looks more square than usual. The square appearance is because the ball of the upper arm bone has been displaced out of the joint socket. It's been forced towards the front of the joint, and also downwards, distorting the normal rounded appearance of the shoulder girdle.

Once this has happened, it's imperative that the player be transported to a medical facility for reduction of the dislocation. During this transportation, I strongly advise that the player be allowed to hold the arm in whatever position he or she feels comfortable with.

No attempt should be made to move the arm into what the player or anyone else thinks is a more natural position. Significant pain and also muscle spasm would be likely, as the body's natural defences signal the inadvisability of the arm being moved

Splint a dislocated finger immediately.

All injuries to the shoulder girdle are potentially serious.

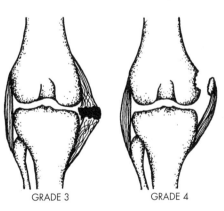

GRADE 1　　GRADE 2　　GRADE 3　　GRADE 4

Grading of ligament injuries, using the knee as an example. This grading applies to all large joints in the body.

> *Further treatment and rehabilitation should be coordinated by a doctor and a physiotherapist before any return to training or competition.*

> *In all codes of football, the injury that the player fears most is an injury to the knee joint.*

in any further direction which could cause damage to the shoulder joint.

The further treatment and rehabilitation of such an injury should be coordinated by a doctor and a physiotherapist before any return to training or competition is contemplated.

Another injury which can occur in the shoulder girdle, particularly in rugby, is damage to the acromio-clavicular joint. This is a small joint in the upper aspect of the shoulder girdle between the collarbone and the acromium (at the top of the shoulder).

These injuries usually result from direct contact to the shoulder girdle. In rugby, this usually occurs in the formation of the scrum.

The more minor injuries to the acromioclavicular joint can be treated with the application of ice and rest for the first 24 to 48 hours. Alternatively, they can be treated by reducing the movement of the arm and using oral anti-inflammatory medications such as Feldene™, Voltaren™ or Naprosyn™.

More significant injuries to this joint may require prolonged periods of rest and rehabilitation with physiotherapy treatment, utilising electrotherapy and specific strengthening exercises for the supporting muscles.

THE DREADED KNEE JOINT INJURIES

In all codes of football, the injury that the player fears most is an injury to the knee joint. There are a variety of injuries which can occur to the knee joint.

Fortunately, less severe injuries usually occur more often than severe ones. Minor injuries usually involve damage to the meniscus.

There are two compartments in the knee joint — the medial (inner compartment) and the lateral (the outer compartment). Each compartment has a meniscus. This cartilaginous disc can be torn, particularly when a player twists or turns suddenly on his or her leg.

This typically happens when the leg is fixed, for example, stuck in mud, or when an opponent is standing on a player's foot. Such a rotation of the knee joint can result in a torn meniscus, which is usually accompanied by some damage to the capsule surrounding the knee joint.

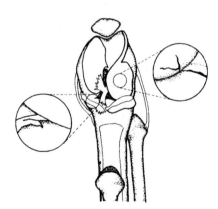

The inside of the knee can be damaged easily in sports involving twisting or pivoting. The damage is usually to either the meniscus, shown on the left, or to the cartilage lining of the joint, as shown on the right.

Damage can also occur to the ligament structures supporting the joint.

The ligaments supporting the knee joint are divided into two groups. The ligaments within the joint itself are the anterior and the posterior cruciate ligaments. The ligaments outside the joint capsule are the medial and lateral collateral ligaments.

Treatment

If the knee joint becomes swollen within the first four hours following injury, it must be assumed that bleeding has occurred within the joint. This may be caused by a fracture to one of the bones within the joint, damage to one of the internal ligaments or the tearing of the meniscus.

If this rapid swelling occurs, immediate medical treatment should be started. If there are delays in providing such treatment, then the application of RICE is strongly recommended until a doctor sees the player.

However, if the swelling in the knee joint occurs slowly, that is, over a 24-hour period, it's usually due to irritation of the synovium — the inner lining under the capsule joint. Such irritation causes an increase in the amount of the fluid normally produced by the synovium. This in turn results in a swelling within the joint.

The problem isn't as urgent as that of rapid swelling in the joint, but the application of RICE is still vitally important. If an improvement doesn't occur within two to three days, then I would recommend you seek medical advice about the best management of the injury.

A major advance in recent years is that doctors can now see the internal aspects of a joint using a procedure known as arthroscopy. An arthroscope is a tiny telescope with a light source. Not only the knee joint, but also the shoulder, ankle and elbow joints can be seen using this procedure.

A small hole is made and an arthroscope is inserted in the joint

The application of RICE is strongly recommended until a doctor sees the player.

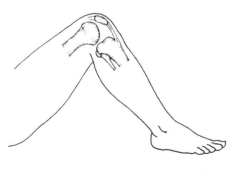

Normal position of the knee bent to 90°.
When there is damage to the posterior cruciate ligament, as happens when the knee is hyperextended, in the 90° position the lower leg falls back.

Injuries to the external ligaments of the knee joint usually occur when a player is twisting or pivoting and then collides with an opponent.

and, through other small holes into the joint, instruments can be inserted and appropriate procedures performed within the joint.

This avoids the need to make a large incision for investigative procedures. Less time is spent in hospital and post-operative rehabilitation is much faster. More significant intervention may be called for with a more major injury to the external or internal ligaments supporting the knee joint.

Injuries to the external ligaments of the knee joint usually occur when a player is twisting or pivoting and then collides with an opponent. The sideways force applied to the outside of the knee joint stresses the inner ligament, the medial collateral ligament.

If the force is applied from the inside aspect of the knee joint, the damage occurs to the outer ligament, the lateral collateral ligament.

It's far more common for the force to be applied from the outside, so a medial collateral ligament injury is the more usual of the two complaints.

A sports medicine doctor typically sees various types or stages of injury, from the more minor, resulting from damage to a small portion of the ligament fibres, to a moderate injury, which typically involves damage to 40 to 60 per cent of the ligament fibres, to a severe injury or a type three injury, which involves more than 60 per cent of the ligament fibres.

Clearly, how serious the injury is determines how unstable the joint will be. This becomes evident upon examination.

In a significant injury to the knee joint involving the ligaments, it's also quite common to see damage to the capsule and nerve endings which supply information to the brain about the knee joint function.

An example comes to mind of a football match when a player received a significant injury to his right knee joint and was taken from the ground. My initial examination showed he had completely disrupted his anterior cruciate ligament and his medial and lateral collateral ligaments. However, he had felt no pain, and in fact, because it was a grand final, was quite keen to return. He actually tried to stand and take a few steps before the knee completely collapsed from under him. It was only then that he realised the full seriousness of the injury to his knee joint. Within half an hour, the knee was swollen and quite painful. But in those initial few minutes following the injury, he was quite oblivious to how serious the

THE VALUE OF NON-STRETCH TAPES

Non-stretch tapes applied to joints may do two things. Firstly, a small amount of mechanical support may be given to ligament structures. Secondly, proprioception (sensory response) may be enhanced. For a full discussion, see page 14.

injury was. He had felt no pain because of the damage which had occurred to the nerve receptors within the capsule of the joint itself.

THE RISK OF SERIOUS INJURIES

Unfortunately, the vigorous nature of contact sports such as football carries the risk of serious injury to the head, the eyes and internal organs such as the lungs, the spleen and kidneys, because of direct forces being applied to the chest and abdomen.

HEAD INJURIES

Closed head injuries (no open cuts but possible internal bruising or bleeding) are quite common in football. They can result in brief unconsciousness. It's therefore important when assessing closed head injuries to inquire if there's been any loss of consciousness, or if the player feels dazed and confused. Establish the player's level of arousal and also whether there's been any short-term memory loss.

Ask simple questions such as:

- What's your name?
- What position were you playing in?
- Which direction were you kicking?
- What stage was the game at when you were injured?
- What's the score?

All these questions are very important in establishing whether he or she has sustained a head injury.

Treatment

If there's concern about a possible head injury, always err on the side of caution, particularly with young players. Immediately remove them from the ground to avoid the risk of further injury and more serious complications.

If the player continues to have symptoms such as sleepiness, difficulty in arousal, the development of nausea and vomiting, then prompt evaluation and observation for at least four to six hours is a must.

My rule when dealing with players involved in contact sports is to ban them from playing contact sports for two to three weeks if they have sustained a closed head injury. This applies even if temporary loss of consciousness hasn't occurred. This safeguard of insisting on a rest period particularly applies to children or young adolescents. Never take risks with possible head injuries.

THE DANGER OF SPINAL INJURIES IN RUGBY

Rugby, because of the nature of the sport, involves the risk of spinal injuries, particularly in the scrum, when players are in position and applying a force straight down the spine. By hitting the head directly or by hitting the shoulder, shock force is applied down the spine.

The danger of spinal injuries was recently highlighted in the United States in gridiron when they had to

Never take risks with head injuries.

Remove an injured player from the ground immediately.

> *In rugby union a player is in a position where the forces generated are like being hit by a small car at 60 km/h.*

make a rule change on a tackle known as 'spearing'. A player tackling an opponent would put his head down (and he had a helmet on to protect him) and actually dive like a spear to hit his opponent. While they might not get too bad a head injury because they were wearing a helmet, the force could travel straight down the head, where the helmet finished, to where the cervical spine created a nice fulcrum to snap about C6 or C7 and result in the victim being a low quadriplegic.

There only have to be one or two of these injuries in high school football, with subsequent court cases and big damages awards, and the incentive for sports administrators to reduce such injury risks becomes obvious. Such injuries can happen all too easily, particularly in rugby union, where a player is in a position where the forces generated are like being hit by a small car at 60 km/h.

While this kind of injury is a problem with all football codes, rugby has a specific problem in the way players tackle and throw opponents to the ground.

Injury prevention

The important point for children's sport is that there must be a very strict application and understanding of the rules by the referee and the administrators. This understanding also applies to parents so they don't start accusing the referee of not having good reasons for holding up a game. I believe there should be very strict rules about the scrum, how it's formed and the age of the players.

The sport poses particular dangers to the cervical spine or the neck and an injury to this area can cause quite catastrophic damage to the spinal cord, resulting in quadriplegia, very high paraplegia or even death.

Treatment

A spinal injury requires urgent medical attention. Such an injury should be suspected if: a patient complains of numbness or pins and needles below the level of the region where the injury is believed to be (for example, below the neck or the shoulders or in the arms, hands, abdomen or legs); if they're unable to move muscle groups in their arms or legs, or if they have pain in the spinal region. Also be suspicious if they have had a severe blow to the forehead or a whiplash-type movement of their neck.

The most important point is NEVER MOVE anyone suspected of having sustained a spinal injury unless under medical supervision. That's the absolute bottom line in using commonsense caution. It should be in capitals and underlined in your mind. Even minor fractures of the vertebrae can lead to quadriplegia or paraplegia if faulty moving techniques produce dislocation of the fractured vertebrae.

> *There must be a very strict application and understanding of the rules.*

CHEST INJURIES TO FOOTBALLERS

Chest injuries due to direct forces being applied are quite common in Australian Rules football and the rugby codes. Fractured ribs can occur and can result in damage to lung and pleural tissues. There is also a possibility of damage to the spleen, which lies under the left diaphragm in the upper part of the left side of the abdomen.

Sometimes it's difficult to assess whether the player has developed a serious internal injury. This is where it's important, if you're a trainer or coach, to know your players — particularly how they respond to injuries. This will sharpen your perception of whether or not they are seriously injured.

Treatment: an example

An example comes to mind of my first match as the club doctor with the Prahran Football Club. During the first quarter, George Stone, who was a very determined player, was involved in a collision with an opponent. George felt some pain on the left side of his chest and upper abdomen. I examined him during the quarter-time interval. During the examination, he was mildly tender over the left mid to lower rib cage. But he was breathing reasonably well with only mild to moderate discomfort. I asked him whether he was able to keep playing. He replied that he was fine and that he wanted to go back the next quarter. By the time I had left the ground and had walked up the stairs to the coach's box, the game had started. When the ball had been bounced, George Stone attempted to run towards it. He immediately stopped and bent over.

When I saw this, I asked the coach was this normal practice for this particular player. He said this was most unusual, so I immediately got George off the field. An examination with a stethoscope indicated that little, or no, air was entering the left side of his chest. I immediately sent him to the local hospital where an X-ray revealed two fractured ribs and a collapsed left lung.

He was in hospital for three days. Within three weeks he had resumed training and played five weeks after the injury.

THE FIRST FEW HOURS ARE VITAL

I cannot stress enough the importance of erring towards caution when dealing with any injury in contact sports, whether it involves a joint, the head, the eyes or internal organs.

The first few hours following the injury are vital. You need to get the appropriate treatment, so as to avoid serious complications. Simple commonsense and basic first aid principles, particularly when dealing with soft tissue, muscle or joint injuries, can significantly aid recovery and prevent more significant

> **STOP**
>
> *Do not move a player with suspected spinal injuries.*

When a player hits the ground hard, cuts and abrasions occur.

secondary problems.

If not dealt with properly, an injury can delay a player's return to normal competition or even permanently restrict the function of the injured part of the body. Functional disability could result in restricting even the normal activities of daily living. So, proceed with caution.

INFECTION: NEVER TAKE CHANCES

As football is mostly played outdoors, when a player hits the ground hard, cuts and abrasions occur.

Unless the skin injury is substantial, it often doesn't become evident until the end of the game when the player notices that an area of skin around the knee or elbow joint has been damaged — usually an abrasion with some minor cuts.

Avoiding infection is the most important factor in treating these injuries. The best policy is always prevention.

A scrubbing brush became the most feared object for many of the players when I was the club doctor with the Prahran Football Club in the Victorian Football Association. It was the most frequently used part of my medical equipment. Once I had established who had developed an abrasion to the skin and to what region of the body, I made a frequent journey into the shower room with my scrubbing brush. Despite howls of protest and unprintable exclamations by the players about the cleanliness of the wound, the vigorous application of the scrubbing brush to the injury was a very efficient way of removing dirt and debris from the wound. It also helped stimulate the blood supply to the region. Once the player had completed his shower, the application of a clean dressing was necessary.

I'm pleased to say that this simple and direct method prevented secondary infection in 99.99 per cent of cases, to the delight of the coach. There's nothing more frustrating to a club than a key player missing several games because of a primary infection of a skin abrasion.

Clearly, if a player has a large cut which doesn't appear to close easily with the application of sticking plaster or bandage, then prompt medical treatment is necessary to adequately close the wound and promote good healing and minimal scar formation.

Depending on the size and position of the wound, it's common for a player to resume training within a few days. But if there is any concern about the wound, I would keep the player out until the stitches have been removed.

With current concern about transferring infections from one person to another through contact from a bleeding wound, strict adherence to the 'Blood Bin' rules is mandatory. Bleeding from a wound must be controlled and the wound

Athletes involved in contact sports should be vaccinated against hepatitis B.

covered, preferably before the player resumes the playing arena.

I strongly recommend that all athletes involved in contact sports or sports with a high risk of exposure to hepatitis B should be vaccinated against hepatitis B, a serious and potentially fatal disease.

HELPFUL HINTS

Prevention

- Make sure that the playing arena is always clear of any dangerous objects such as protruding sprinkler systems. Check that the goal posts are padded and the boundary line is well away from any fences or cars parked around the arena.
- Make sure the players' equipment is well fitting and in good working order. This includes boots, checking that there are no sharp nails protruding from the stops and that nylon studs haven't worn down excessively.
- Be sure that each player is flexible and has had a good pre-season training session to develop muscle strength and joint mobility and acquire the necessary skills for the game.
- It's very important that players, club officials, umpires and referees understand all the rules governing the game. This will go a long way towards reducing injury risks.

Treatment

- Always err on the side of caution when dealing with injuries to the head, chest, abdomen, joints and muscles. When in doubt, seek medical advice.
- The first four to six hours following any injury are vital to maximise benefits of treatment and minimise serious complications.
- The cornerstone of any treatment in contact sports for injuries involving muscles, ligaments or joints is RICE.

CHAPTER 5

BAT AND BALL SPORTS: CRICKET, BASEBALL, SOFTBALL AND FIELD HOCKEY

There's always a risk when children play sports that involve the use of hard balls. However, serious injuries can be minimised with the appropriate protective equipment and a keen understanding of the rules.

BALLS

In sports like cricket, baseball and field hockey, the hardness of the ball should be reduced with younger children, allowing them to enjoy participation in such sports without the fear of being hurt. Rather than have young children play these sports with a lot of protective equipment, use softer balls, particularly in cricket and baseball, until they get older and participate at a more competitive level. Fortunately, in softball the ball is relatively soft. Even so, if thrown at a high speed it can cause considerable bruising and damage to skin and underlying soft tissues. It can even cause broken bones if it hits an extremity such as an extended finger.

In the United States and now in Australia there has been a ball designed for baseball and cricket called the 'IncrediBall' which has a specially-designed softer inner core but has not lost the normal characteristics of either a baseball or cricket ball. The 'IncrediBall' significantly reduces the incidence of serious facial, head and hand injuries, and is now the official ball endorsed by the Victorian Cricket Association for all ages under 12 years.

PROTECTIVE EQUIPMENT

All equipment should be suited to the size, strength and ability of the child.

Batting gloves can be useful. A cricket or baseball striking a batter's fingers can damage the soft tissues and bones. Choose the right sort of gloves — right-handed gloves for those who bat right-handed or else proper left-handed gloves.

In field hockey and cricket shinpads help minimise injuries to the lower leg from the ball or an indiscriminate swing from an opponent's stick.

Groin protectors for boys are appropriate in cricket, baseball, softball and field hockey because an ill-directed ball can cause considerable damage. For adolescent girls, special bras with breast protection may also help prevent serious bruising, particularly when batting in cricket, softball and baseball.

Helmets

I don't believe young children should wear the specialised helmets and face protectors that older adolescents and adults wear for senior cricket. Visors across the face can actually restrict rather than improve a young player's ability to see the ball.

If a protective helmet is to be worn by older children for batting (in cricket and baseball) and close-in fielding I recommend a helmet without a faceguard or visor. Use a firm helmet, similar to that worn by baseballers, which particularly protects the temple area.

Using softer balls and avoiding short-pitched deliveries which rise up towards the head are other practical ways of avoiding serious face or head injuries.

Footwear

Proper footwear is vital in reducing skin injuries involving the soles of the feet and around the toes. High-cut boots for cricketers, particularly bowlers, greatly reduce the risk of ankle sprains. For fast bowlers, or those who are on their feet and are bowling for long periods, shock-absorbing insoles of Sorbathane™ can significantly reduce stress placed on the joints of the lumbar spine, therefore reducing the incidence of spinal stress fractures.

Make Sure it Fits

Parents often overlook the fact that if the equipment isn't the right size, or is otherwise uncomfortable, players won't use it. Lack of thought in selecting the right equipment is a recipe for disaster, as serious injuries can occur if the basic items of safety gear are not worn.

Training

Net practice

Make sure protective netting is in good condition. All practice sessions should be supervised by a teacher or coach. Allow only the batter inside

Use softer balls, the right sort of gloves, and proper footwear.

All practice sessions should be supervised by a teacher or coach.

Make sure bowlers do not bowl unless the net is clear and the batter is ready.

the net, unless you are doing wicketkeeping practice. Allow a maximum of four bowlers to one net. Make sure bowlers do not bowl unless the net is clear and the batter is ready. When someone is bowling, balls should not be collected from inside the net. Bowlers should always face battters so they can see any balls hit in the air.

ENVIRONMENT

Use sunburn cream and hats in all weather conditions. Ensure players drink water before and during the game to prevent dehydration. In hot weather, fluid intake may need to be more frequent. On cooler summer days, an hourly drinks break should be sufficient.

DON'T FORGET THE WARM-UP

All these sports involve a lot of running, twisting and turning. Apart from injuries to bones and joints, and stress fractures, players are liable to sustain ankle sprains, and the commonly-seen strains of the calf, hamstring, and quadriceps muscles in the legs, and other strains to the lower extremities.

It's therefore important for players to warm up adequately before

STRETCHING FOR BASEBALL AND SOFTBALL

Stretching exercises are vital. They prepare the muscles and joints, improve performance and decrease the risk of injury. There are two easy steps to follow. First, the warm-up: six laps around the boundaries. Secondly, stretching: follow diagrams (hold each stretch when you feel mild tension). Hold each stretch for 10 seconds. Repeat 5 times. Stretch when warm, and always stretch before and after activity.

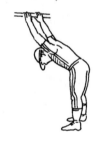

1 Drop your body as the knees bend.

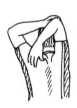

2 Gently pull your elbow behind your head. Repeat with other arm.

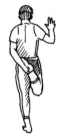

3 Clasp your foot behind your body with alternate hand. Repeat with other leg.

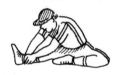

4 Bend forward from the hips toward one foot. Repeat with other leg.

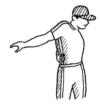

5 Hold onto a wall or door. Turn your head to look over your left shoulder. Repeat with other arm.

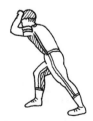

6 Place your rear foot one step from a wall. Point your toes straight ahead. Stretch rear leg. Repeat with other

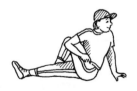

7 Turn your head and upper body to the left. Balance with the elbow on the knee. Repeat with other side.

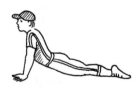

8 Lie on your stomach, hands next to shoulders. Gently push up, keeping your hips flat.

entering the sporting arena.

The warm-up should include a stretching program specifically for the muscle groups in the legs and muscle groups around the shoulders, elbows and wrist joints. This significantly helps minimise muscle strain from overstress.

Injury prevention

In field hockey, the strict application of the rule not allowing players to swing their sticks above shoulder height is very important in minimising the serious facial or head injuries which can occur in the more heated moments of the game.

It's also important in cricket, baseball and softball that there's strict adherence to the rules to avoid particularly serious facial or head injuries when the ball is intentionally thrown towards an opponent. Many nasty injuries can result, particularly to the face and eyes.

As bat and ball sports are usually played on outdoor fields, it's important to carefully check the field and remove any objects thoughtlessly left lying about.

Make sure that the boundary lines are drawn, and clearly mark the field edges. Boundaries should always be well away from large immovable objects (such as fences, posts or sheds) that players can run into when they are intently watching the ball — or an opponent coming at them! Simply following these rules will help to avoid serious bone and internal injuries.

Injuries

When the ball — or on occasions the bat or stick — hits a player, it most commonly bruises the skin and the underlying soft tissues without actually breaking the skin. More severe bruising may be caused to the underlying muscle.

Treatment

Apply ice to the affected area as soon as possible, using either crushed ice in a wet towel or one of the commercially available ice packs. When applying these commercial ice packs, place a wet towel between the ice pack and the skin to avoid burning.

It's vital to reduce swelling, both the initial swelling caused by bleeding under the skin if small blood vessels have been damaged, and the later swelling due to the fluid that accumulates as an inflammatory response to soft tissue injury.

Apply ice for about 20 minutes, every three or four hours over the next 24 hours. This will significantly reduce swelling and any extensive scarring that may occur to the soft tissue because of fluid build-up.

Rest the injured area, particularly for the first 24 to 48 hours. This promotes maximum healing as blood is diverted from the active muscles to the area where the injury has occurred.

Commonsense and basic first aid can make a big difference to recovery rates.

Apply ice as soon as possible to a bruise.

If an extremity such as a finger has been damaged, apply a splint with a bandage to rest the area for a few days. Where the bruising involves deeper structures, particularly the muscles, then the period of splinting may have to be prolonged and also the application of ice may be extended for two or three days.

It's important to resume movement of the injured area as soon as the pain has been reduced, to avoid stiffness of the joints above or below the damaged area. Begin movement slowly, within the limitations of pain, with a slow, stretching program for the injured muscles.

Damage to bones and joints

Sometimes it's very difficult to establish whether an underlying bone has also been damaged. This is particularly true of the forearm and hand, where there's very little soft tissue padding between skin and bone.

Treatment

If there's an obvious deformity in the alignment of the bones and the injury is not in an area where there's a joint, assume there's a broken bone. Splint the area and transport the player to a hospital or medical facility for X-rays.

If the damaged area involves a joint and there's a deformity when compared with the corresponding body part on the other side, the injury may be either a fracture or a dislocation of the joint. Immediately get the involved limb or joint into a comfortable position and apply a splint if possible. Send the player promptly for X-rays and other appropriate medical treatment.

Sometimes a ball, bat or stick may hit a forearm and cause what appears to be a contusion. However, as the forearm bones can be very close to the skin, it may be a fracture even though there's no sign of deformity. So be alert and err on the side of caution.

'Spot-on' diagnosis

I well remember making a wrong diagnosis when I was medical officer for the Victorian Cricket Team. It was late on the second day of a match being played at the Junction Oval between Victoria and Western Australia. Victoria was in trouble, having lost two early wickets, then Graham Yallop was struck a nasty blow on the right forearm from a short-pitched delivery from Mick Malone.

Before I went out to the crease to inspect Yallop's injury, the Victorian team captain, John Scholes, emphasised the importance of Yallop continuing to bat. Yallop was in considerable pain when I examined his arm. There was a tender area over the mid-portion of the forearm but no obvious deformity.

I told him that he had probably just sustained some deep bruising and advised him to keep batting. As I returned to the dressing room, he

Immediately immobilise a fracture.

drove the next ball from Malone for four runs, and I felt quite pleased with my decision to keep him batting.

At the end of the day's play, 40 minutes later, I examined Yallop's arm again in the dressing room. Because it was quite tender over the ulna, which is one of the forearm bones, I decided he should have an X-ray just to make sure it wasn't broken.

To my surprise, there was a fracture through the ulna which was undisplaced, and Yallop had to have his right arm immobilised in a plaster cast for the next six weeks. I was henceforth nicknamed 'SPOT ON', a facetious reference to my accuracy in diagnosing this injury.

Rotator cuff lesion

In cricket, softball and baseball, throwing or bowling can place excessive stress on the shoulder and elbow joints. This action, although varying from a bent arm throw in baseball to bowling overarm with a straight arm in cricket and throwing the ball underarm when pitching in softball, can cause stress resulting in damage to the capsules and ligaments which support the joints.

Also, the outfielders and infielders in these three sports can also sustain injuries to the elbow and shoulder joints, particularly when attempting to throw the ball either a long distance or very quickly back to another fieldsman.

Shoulder joint injury

A common shoulder joint injury occurs in the tendons of those muscles that perform rotation movements. This is known as a 'rotator cuff lesion'. This may be either a tearing of the combined tendon of four small muscles at the shoulder joint or irritation of one or more of the tendons, also known as 'tenosynovitis' or 'tendonitis'.

Rotator cuff lesion can result in thickening of the tendon. Difficulty then arises when the tendon has to move through a small bony canal in the shoulder joint when rotating the arm or lifting it up from the side. This is called a shoulder impingement.

Treatment

The best treatment should involve rest from the sporting activity until pain and irritation subside. Apply ice to the

In cricket, softball and baseball, throwing or bowling can place excessive stress on the shoulder and elbow joints.

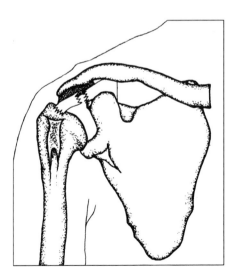

Rotator cuff lesions. Either inflammation or tearing can occur in this area of the shoulder.

The best treatment involves rest.

shoulder joint. Analgesics and anti-inflammatory medication may be needed to ease excessive discomfort. Seek medical advice if the irritation in the shoulder girdle doesn't resolve itself over 10 to 14 days with rest and ice.

Elbow joint injury

Irritation to the elbow joint is a common injury for fielders who throw the ball fairly regularly or very hard, and also for baseball pitchers.

The many different problems that can occur at the elbow include strains of the muscles around the elbow joint, inflammation of the medial or lateral epicondyle, fractures of the elbow joint bones, and the development of spurs and degenerative changes in the joint.

In the 1960s, the development of the Pee Wee League in the United States lead to an epidemic of elbow problems. Stress placed on the elbow by the pitching action has since been found to be the cause of multiple pathological conditions collectively known as 'Little Leaguer's Elbow'.

A player with Little Leaguer's Elbow usually complains of pain and, as a result, may be unable to throw. The pain can be generalised around the elbow joint because of the different areas that can be irritated. There may be some swelling, and prolonged activity can produce stiffness in the joint which decreases the range of movement.

Most cases of elbow joint pain can be successfully treated with rest.

Watching for signs and symptoms of elbow problems will greatly improve the chances of early diagnosis and treatment.

Treatment

Most cases of elbow pain caused by excessive pitching can be successfully treated by rest and, if necessary, by splinting. Anti-inflammatory medication and the application of ice may also be necessary in more resistant cases.

However, prevention is the best treatment of all. The Little League has rules that limit the amount a child may pitch during a game. And, in the very young baseball league, known here as Tee Ball, there's no pitching at all. The players just hit the ball off a tee.

This has significantly reduced the incidence of serious or permanent damage occurring to the elbow joint until Little Leaguers reach an age where the elbow muscle can effectively support the elbow joint. Recent recommendations further limit the amount of throwing allowed and prevent curve-ball pitching and other more difficult pitches.

Unfortunately, there's no limitation on pitching at home and during practice. Therefore parents and coaches should be aware of the risks. Watching for signs and symptoms of elbow problems will greatly improve the chances of early diagnosis and treatment.

Good judgement and conservative measures are vital in preventing significant deformities and impairment of the elbow joint function.

STRESS FRACTURES

Stress fractures in the lumbar region of the spine are common in adolescents. They may even go unnoticed, unless the individual puts a strain on the lower back and requires an X-ray of this region.

Fast bowlers in cricket often suffer stress fractures in the spine. We only have to look at such bowlers as Dennis Lillee, Rodney Hogg, Bruce Reid and Dennis Hickey to understand the stresses fast bowling places on the lumbar spine.

Stress fractures in the spine are difficult to treat because they are difficult to diagnose. The player may have a vague sort of back pain. Any unexplained back pain is always significant in a young adolescent who plays an active sport such as cricket or basketball. A stress fracture should always be suspected.

A bone scan will usually show up a stress fracture. A bone scan is like an X-ray except that it involves injecting a radio-nuclear dye, which then concentrates in areas of new bone growth or where bone has been laid down (as occurs in a fracture site).

A computerised tomography X-ray (CT scan) may also be used to specifically diagnose the problem.

Stress fractures are difficult to treat. The simple answer is that rest is possibly the best treatment of all. In the early days of the injury, the patient should rest and avoid stressing factors on the spine. Following that period of rest, a suitable exercise program will build up fitness and promote a full recovery. An appropriate rest time would vary greatly, but for a fast bowler this could well be a whole season.

GUIDELINES FOR FAST BOWLERS

According to recent studies, young fast bowlers are the players most prone to injury.

WARM-UPS

I recommend these minimum requirements for fast bowlers aged 11 to 13.

Upper body strength: more than 30 push-ups in one minute

Aerobic fitness: more than 3000 m in a 15-minute run

Sit and reach flexibility: more than + 5 cm

Abdominal strength: more than 30 sit-ups in one minute

PHYSICAL DEMAND

Practice should consist of two 30-minute bowling sessions each week (for players under 13). Matches should involve two spells of four overs each (for players under 13). Limit the number of matches to no more than one per week. Limit the practice time of bowlers playing for more than one team.

> **STOP**
> Don't ignore back pain.

> *Stress fractures in the spine are difficult to treat because they are difficult to diagnose.*

FAST BOWLING TECHNIQUE

SIX FUNDAMENTALS OF BOWLING9

These guidelines assume a right-handed bowler. The opposite would apply for left-handed bowlers.

SIDE-ON TECHNIQUE

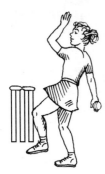

1 Run-up
The approach should be at the best speed for the individual. However, this must allow the bowler time to adopt a side-on position at delivery. Speed should increase gradually, culminating in optimal speed about three or four strides before delivery.

2 Back foot
Place the rear foot parallel to the bowling crease.

3 Impact
Chest and hips should face the bowler's stumps.
Shoulder and hips point toward the batter until just before the ball is thrown.
Thrust the non-bowling arm high into the air.
Look behind the front arm without arching the back.

4 Delivery stride
Elbow of the non-bowling arm accelerates into the side of the body.
There should be lateral flexion and extension of the spine, without arching and twisting of the spine.
Front leg should land pointing straight down the wicket or slightly to the on-side for a right handed batter, aligned with the back foot.

5 Release
Bend the knee of the front leg slightly, to absorb some of the impact.

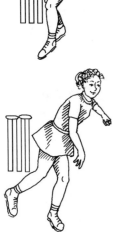

6 Follow-through
Bowling arm follows through diagonally downwards and backwards (past the outside left leg for a right-handed bowler).
Continue for at least six steps after throwing of the ball to gradually reduce forward momentum.

FRONT-ON TECHNIQUE

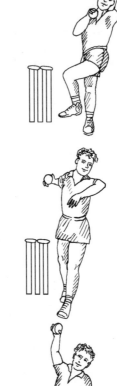

This technique is used by West Indian bowlers.

1 Run-up
The approach should be at the best speed for the individual.

2 Back foot
Place the rear foot pointing straight down the wicket or slightly towards the on-side, that is the fine leg position for a right handed batter.

3 Impact
Chest and hips should face the batter.
Thrust the non-bowling arm high into the air.
Look straight down the wicket, on the inside of the non-bowling arm.

4 Delivery stride
Point the front leg when landing straight down the wicket.
Shoulders should be parallel to the crease.
The elbow of the non-bowling arm accelerates downwards.
The bowler's arm should lead the forward movement of the body.

5 Release
Bend the knee of the front leg slightly to absorb some of the impact.

6 Follow-through
Bowling arm follows down the side of the body.
Continue for at least six steps after throwing the ball to gradually reduce forward momentum.

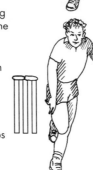

IMPORTANT NOTE

Coaches should ensure that fast bowlers use either the side-on technique or the front-on technique (if they have sufficient shoulder flexibility), not a combination of these techniques.

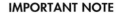

HELPFUL HINTS

Always make sure that the playing field is clear of any objects and that the boundaries of the playing field are well away from fences and other immovable objects.

Protective equipment should be used. For example, batting gloves, groin protectors (in girls, breast protection), in field hockey, correctly-fitting shinpads. If a firmer ball is being used, then a protective helmet may be necessary when batting in cricket and baseball.

Overall, it's important that there is appropriate and consistent application of the rules in all of these bat and ball sports. Commonsense by umpires and administrators can significantly reduce traumatic injuries such as those which occur as a result of high-pitched balls in cricket.

The wearing of proper footwear is important in reducing skin injuries involving the soles of the feet and around the toes. Also, high-cut boots in cricket, particularly for bowlers, greatly reduce the risk of ankle sprains.

Always err on the side of caution if concerned about any injury. Suspect a fracture if there's any deformity or significant pain or swelling, even after the application of ice. Seek medical advice as soon as possible.

Overuse injuries classically occur in the shoulders and elbows of baseballers and softballers and in the mid to lower back in cricket.

Preventive measures should include using Sorbathane™ in shoes and restricting a young bowler to no more than 6 to 10 overs, and 10 to 14 overs in young adolescents.

CHAPTER 6

Water sports: swimming, surfing, water-skiing and sailing

Swimming has one big advantage over other sports. Water buoyancy reduces gravity by 60 to 70 per cent, so swimmers don't stress their lower back and other weight-bearing joints as do runners and jumpers.

Many of the problems young swimmers encounter are caused by a combination of endurance and speed, and discrepancies between swimmers' muscle development and the performance expectations of their coach and parents. By the time hard training starts, they have started their growth spurt. However, because of the difference in the growth rates of different tissues, their bones grow faster and get stronger earlier than their muscles.

It takes *12 to 18 months* for the strength and stretch of the muscles to catch up to the bone strength and length. This disparity puts a lot of pressure on the muscles — in swimming or any other sport.

Growth spurts

Girls start maturing earlier than boys and have a very rapid growth spurt. Boys usually catch up around the ages of 16 to 18. This means than an 11- or 12-year-old girl can be very much stronger than a boy of the same age. At this age, a girl can usually produce greater physical effort and sustain it for a longer period than a boy. There are exceptions, of course. Some boys start their growth earlier and are stronger earlier. In general, however, girls have the edge, which explains why they compete very early in swimming and gymnastics.

Muscle strain injuries

Muscle strain affecting the upper torso into the shoulder region is the most common type of injury for swimmers, along with tenosynovitis. Swimmers strain muscles around their shoulderblades, in their shoulders and their upper arms.

They also get muscle strains further down and, of course, muscle strains in their thighs and buttocks.

Treatment

Treatment involves applying RICE for 24 to 48 hours, followed by simple stretching manoeuvres (see page 9).

EYE INFECTIONS

Children who swim regularly in pools often suffer eye irritations from chlorinated or salt-chlorinated pools. There are excellent goggles which young swimmers who do a lot of swimming can wear to avoid eye irritations.

I believe goggles are now so good that they should always be used in sea water, too. It's easy to get eye infections from sea water when swimming near drains emptying alongside beaches. The drains are often partly concealed, so you may not even realise a potential hazard exists.

Treatment

It's important that eye infections are properly diagnosed. One of the best sayings is: beware of the unilateral red eye. This means a red eye on the one side and not on the other. The inflammation and redness can be due to a foreign body in the eye. Accordingly, such symptoms should always ring bells that there may be a bit of dirt, grit or even a piece of glass in the eye which could be causing the infection. No amount of antibiotics will get rid of the foreign body.

Almost invariably, if an athlete gets an infection in one eye, it crosses to the other side. So if they have bilateral red eyes, it's usually due to an irritation or infection. The best treatment is to keep the eyes clean and use antibiotic eye-drops.

If the eye is really irritated, you should apply an eye pad to rest the eye and every two hours apply the drops. In a day or two, it usually clears up. Medical advice should be sought about an eye infection which doesn't settle down.

Don't keep eye-drops for too long because they have a limited effective life. It's a good idea to keep them in the fridge. Once the infection has cleared up, throw the drops away because bugs can grow in the eye-drops over a period of time.

EAR INFECTIONS

Ear infections are also a common problem — particularly from swimming in public pools. If children complain of earache, and if there's no external sign of ear infection, have them checked immediately by your local family GP or an Ear, Nose and Throat specialist.

Glue ears

Many children have problems with what is called 'glue ears', a build-up of fluid behind the ear drum (the tympanic membrane). The fluid is so

---

Seek medical advice if an eye or ear infection doesn't settle down.

Keep ear- and eye-drops in the fridge and don't keep them for too long.

> **THROW AWAY OLD MEDICINES**
>
> It's a little-realised fact about eye-drops or ear-drops that the solution in which the antibody is held is also an ideal medium for growing bacteria.
>
> Therefore it's very important to keep the drops in the fridge and not to hold on to them once the expiry date is reached or the infection has cleared up. Otherwise, a few months later when your child has another eye or ear infection and you use the old bottle, you will be putting drops now full of germs into your child's eyes or ears.

Sterilise ear plugs in hot water every few weeks.

thick that it doesn't drain away into the back of the throat. This is a middle-ear infection and may not be caused by swimming. The child may simply have ear problems which need treatment. Initially, try medication to drain the fluid away. In chronic cases, this won't always work. It's then appropriate to insert grommets (little tubes) into the ear drum. This increases the pressure which helps drain the gunky material down through the throat. While this solves one problem, it sometimes creates another. Once the tubes have been put in, a connection is established between the external environment and the middle ear which was previously protected by a membrane.

Ear plugs

If the child goes swimming, fluid can flow straight through into the middle ear and cause further infection.

The best way to avoid this is to get special earplugs made. The plugs fit snugly into the ears. Children as young as four can learn to fit their own plugs. Some parents put Blu-Tac™ into their children's ears as well as getting them to wear a rubber swimming cap. Blu-Tac is a good, cheap method of plugging up the ear if your children are getting a lot of external ear infections from the swimming pool. There are now other similar materials on the market as well, which are for use as a putty material to insert into the external ear canal.

Children should not, of course, share the Blu-Tac, because there is a risk of cross-infections. I would recommend earplugs be sterilised in hot water every few weeks and kept in their own little containers. Children will respond well if they are taught how to use the plugs properly and realise they are not things to play with. It becomes a conditioned reflex to wear their plugs whenever they go swimming or even get into the bath.

EQUIPMENT

Goggles: to protect the eyes from chlorine, especially when involved in regular training.

Ear plugs: to prevent 'swimmer's ear' when involved in regular training.

Nose clips: for those swimmers (especially backstrokers) with ear problems.

Weights: can be used in training to help the developing swimmer, but monitor programs carefully. Do not introduce them too early. You need a good balance between muscle development and flexibility, with the workload increasing gradually. Otherwise injury can result from straining or overuse of muscles.

SURFING: COMMONSENSE NOT OVERCONFIDENCE

INJURY PREVENTION

The most important thing in prevention of surfing injuries is to surf in a safe area. No matter how great the surf looks, beware — there may be very dangerous rips, concealed reefs and unknown undertows. Wherever possible, children should always swim at a beach patrolled by lifesavers. This is ignored by numerous people of all age groups. Every year, good samaritans drown going to the rescue of swimmers in trouble at unpatrolled beaches. Lifesavers have hundreds of examples a year of near-misses where they have to make rescues in treacherous stretches of surf clearly outside the marked flags.

Even when swimming in a patrolled area of beach, teach children not to overlook the tried and proven buddy system. Having someone with them can make the difference for those few vital minutes until lifesavers can reach them. Cramps are just as unpredictable as dangerous undertows. No one is immune!

Also, children should not be allowed to go surfing unless they are very strong swimmers. If they are out in very difficult swimming conditions, the slightest problem (such as a sudden wind change) could mean the child is a kilometre offshore before you know it. Overconfidence can be fatal. Stark and horrifying statistics confirm this every year.

Surf in a safe area.

SURF SAFETY TIPS

- Make sure your child is a strong swimmer and can swim unaided for at least 30 minutes.
- Ensure that he or she wears an ankle strap. The ankle strap attached to the board and to the surfer's ankle stops the board from shooting out of control and possibly hitting either the rider or an unsuspecting swimmer.
- Impress on your child the importance of always surfing in areas patrolled by lifesavers — no matter how tempting the surf looks elsewhere.

Ankle straps should always be worn.

Teach children to always surf or swim with someone — use the buddy system.

Ankle straps

When surfboard riding, ankle straps should always be used. Apart from the hassle of having to chase the board after falling off, the most important reason for wearing an ankle strap is to avoid head injuries. A surprising amount of damage can be caused by the point end of the board and the fin at the back when the board goes flying through the air in vigorous surf. With boogie board riding, wrist straps should be used for the same reasons.

The strange thing is that the stray board seems to have the habit of hitting the rider more than the innocent bystander. An interesting study in California found that about 75 per cent of all head injuries to surfers were caused by their own boards! Typically, the board goes straight up and then straight down while the rider who has fallen off is being bounced around in the surf. While the people around can see the board flying and have time to get out of the way, the rider who has lost the board tends to come straight up just as the board is coming straight down!

Water-skiing and Sailing

There are three basic rules for safe water-skiing and sailing:

1 Children must be able to swim well.

2 They must be adequately trained in how to water-ski and sail.

3 They must wear safety vests.

Endurance swimming

I think that all children should be able to swim constantly for at least 30 minutes. You simply don't know what can happen and I think that children should be good swimmers before advancing to more ambitious water activities. Endurance swimming is of vital importance and should be encouraged by parents, swimming water-skiing organisations.

Training

When water-skiing, always be conscious of the danger of snags in dams, lakes and rivers with dead trees just under the surface. It is also essential that you have a very good driver who knows what he or she is doing. First of all, there's the risk of running into other people. Secondly, it's easy to do the wrong thing when a surprise situation suddenly confronts you.

Next, take the time to know your water-skiers. How good are they and how quickly can you pull them out of the water? This particularly applies to your children's friends who may be out for the day with you.

Have an observer facing the water-skier at all times (not looking the other way, like the driver). The observer can then efficiently tell the driver to slow down or stop if the water-skier is having problems. There's no other way for the water-skier to communicate to the driver that he or she is in real trouble.

So it's important that you should have an experienced driver working with a good observer, and without a lot of distractions. Avoid having a boat full of people.

Alcohol is an absolute 'no-no'. It causes more trouble than anything else. Fuzzed coordination and slow reactions are an invitation for trouble.

SAFETY VESTS

It really upsets me to see children water-skiing or sailing without safety vests. I suppose for some children it's more important to look good than to wear wimpish things like safety vests but it should be a rule, in every family, that no child goes water-skiing or sailing unless he or she is wearing a safety vest.

For sailors, there's always the danger of being hit by the boom, temporarily dazed and knocked overboard. I have first-hand experience of this. Sailing with my cousins, I was once hit by the boom and almost knocked out. I woke up floating in the briny. The vest had kept my head up and saved me from certain drowning.

INJURIES

Injuries to water-skiers are mainly shoulder soreness and back problems because of the pulling on the rope, particularly with novice skiers.

The most serious injuries occur when falling off at speed, running into a bank or hitting an underwater snag. All of these are totally avoidable. You can have pleasurable water-skiing with minimal injuries if the basic safety factors are heeded.

THE DANGERS OF HYPOTHERMIA

A word of caution about hypothermia (abnormally low body temperature). I wrote earlier (in the Guidelines for Running section) about the dangers of small children running too vigorously in hot weather and the risks of dehydration and hyperthermia. Children become hypothermic much more quickly than adults.

This means they can die fairly rapidly, depending on the clothes they are wearing, how cold the water is, the wind-chill factor, how well they swim and how well they can support themselves if they are not using a good lifejacket or have no lifejacket at all.

The factor which works in children's favour is that their cardiovascular system can sustain much greater changes to their pulse rate and blood pressure. A good example of this was the recent case of the young child in the United States who fell into a frozen canal and was under the water for between 10 and 15 minutes. He was floppy and blue

Children become hypothermic quickly, but their cardiovascular systems can sustain great changes.

and almost dead when rescuers pulled him out but his system had shut down so effectively that he was able to survive without long-term damage.

'Shut down' means that there are certain priorities which the body gives for its blood supply. Skin is the least of them. Then there's muscle and the intestines and other areas such as the kidneys. The body tries to give maximum protection to the vessels and the arteries to the brain and heart. They are the very last things the body shuts down. The body does the best it can to preserve the brain function because once the brain dies, everything dies. It's better to lose a few fingers or even limbs than to lose the brain!

Children have a greater ability to cope with this shut-down period than older people because of the state of their heart, their coronary vessels and the vessels to their brain.

INJURIES IN SWIMMING

Swimming is a non-contact sport so those injuries which do occur usually result from using a specific muscle or joint excessively (overuse injuries).

LAY TERM	MEDICAL TITLE	SYMPTONS AND SIGNS	PRINCIPLES OF MANAGEMENT	PRINCIPLES OF PREVENTION
Swimmer's ear	Otitis externa	Pain in ear, itching	Anti-fungal ear drops	Attention to drying out ears; ear plugs
Irritated eyes		Pain and itching of eye	Eye drops	Goggles
Swimmer's shoulder	Supraspinatus Tendonitis	Painful arc of movement; tender over tendon; pain on resisted abduction	Rest, ice, anti-inflammatory drugs; physiotherapy; training modification	Warm-up, stretching; gradual increase in training; variation in training
Breastroker's knee	1. Medical ligament strain	Local tenderness; pain on stressing medial ligament	Physiotherapy; training modification; attention to stroke/kick	Slow increase in training load; variation in training
	2. Patello-femoral pain	Pain on squatting, on stairs; tenderness around patella	Physiotherapy—McConnell technique	

TRUNK-STRENGTHENING EXERCISES ARE VERY IMPORTANT IN THE WARM-UP

1(a)

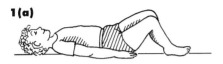

1(a) Lie on your back with knees together and bent. Place feet flat on the floor. Keeping your shoulders still, rock knees slowly to the right and then

1(b)

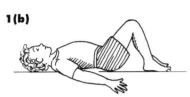

1(b) to the left.

2(a)

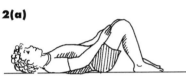

2(a) Start as for exercise 1. Place hands on front of thighs and keep feet flat on the floor.

2(b)

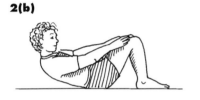

2(b) Lift head and shoulders, sliding hands towards knees. Lower. Be careful not to flex the spine too far: do not do a full sit-up. Keep your hands above your knees. Starting with your knees a little straighter makes this exercise harder.

3

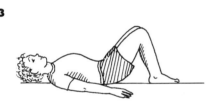

3 Start as for exercise 1. Keep your buttocks and shoulders touching the floor at all times. Tighten your stomach muscles, tuck your seat up and flatten the small of your back onto the floor. Relax. Then roll onto your seat and arch the hollow at the base of your spine. Tilt the pelvis, not the rib cage.

4

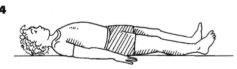

4 Lie flat on your back, keeping your legs parallel and straight. Push right leg along the floor as though you were making it longer than the left. Hitch the left hip up towards the shoulder. Relax. Repeat with the other leg.

5

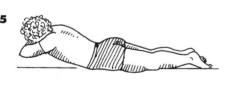

5 Lie on your stomach, resting your forehead on your hands. Lift up arms and head. You may find this very difficult at first but only a few centimetres of elevation are necessary. With practice, you can lift up the legs at the same time.

6

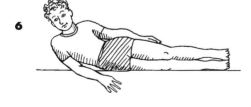

6 Lie on your side. Lift your chest off the floor for a few centimetres and hold. Repeat for the other side.

Water Sports

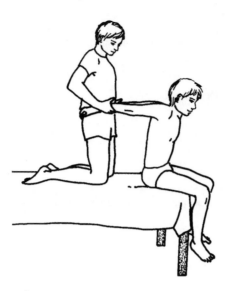

Stretching of adductor muscles of both shoulder joints. These are important for swimmers and throwers.

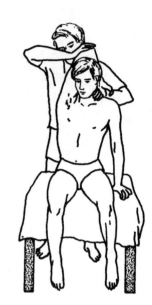

HELPFUL HINTS

- Do an adequate warm-up with slow stretching exercises.
- Guard against eye and ear infections. Always use good goggles and earplugs when swimming for long periods.
- Avoid overtraining and overstress, both physical and psychological, especially with young swimmers doing heavy training sessions in the early mornings, before school.
- Muscle strains and joint ligament injuries are common, especially involving the shoulders, upper back and torso. Treatment should involve the reduction of training, RICE and aspirin when necessary, followed by an exercise program.
- People who water-ski, surf and/or windsurf should be good swimmers.
- Check all equipment to make sure it's in good working order.
- Know the waters you're skiing or surfing on and follow all local instructions and safety suggestions.

CHAPTER 7

BMX BIKE RIDING, SKATEBOARDING, ROLLERBLADING, HORSE RIDING, SNOW-SKIING AND ICE SKATING

While horse riding is very popular in Australia because of the broad expanses of our countryside and our English background, the riding sports which are really booming are BMX racing, skateboarding and rollerblading.

RIDING SAFE ON THE STREETS

MAINTENANCE

Several recent surveys in New South Wales and Victoria have revealed the alarmingly poor state of repair of schoolchildren's bicycles. Poor brakes, tyres and rust-weakened frames are the common trouble spots.

Take a close look at your son or daughter's bike and you could be jolted into doing something. Your apathy today could mean your child going under a truck or bus tomorrow.

Accidents don't always happen to other people. Every day, there are hundreds of near-misses for children on bikes on Australian roads.

SIZE

Check that your child's bike is suited to him/her. An amazing number of children ride hand-me-down bikes which are too big for them. An unsteady child on a bicycle is often a recipe for disaster on crowded roads, with today's deadline pressures pushing truckies, bus drivers and motorists alike.

FLAGS AND BELLS

A flag is one of the best safety features available for young children riding 30 cm (12 inch) and 40 cm (16 inch) bikes, which are otherwise hard to see in streets lined with parked cars. A tall orange safety flag gives an excellent high profile for cycling children, making them immediately

A tall orange safety flag gives an excellent high profile for cycling children.

Helmets should bear the SAA logo.

stand out above parked cars. The price (around $76.50, in 1994) is low if it helps prevent your child being knocked off the bike when, sooner or later, he or she does the wrong thing. A loud bicycle-bell is also an excellent addition.

Helmets

The Victorian and NSW governments are to be congratulated on their campaign to get children and adults to wear helmets. The important thing about helmets is that they should bear the SAA logo. This means they have been stringently tested by the Standards Association of Australia. This standard is frequently reviewed to see what further improvements are needed.

One of the authors of this book, Peter Fitzgerald, ran a campaign with articles in the *Melbourne Herald* from March 1980 over four years. He worked with Professor Frank McDermott of the Road Trauma Committee of the Royal Australasian College of Surgeons, the Bicycle Institute of Victoria, schoolteachers and bereaved parents to popularise the use of helmets for child cyclists. The Victorian government subsequently introduced a subsidy scheme to make an SAA-approved helmet an attractive alternative Christmas present to an electronic game.

The then Victorian transport minister, Mr Steve Crabb, deserves credit for that breakthrough — it has put SAA-approved helmets on the heads of more than 100,000 schoolchildren to date. NSW deserves credit for taking up the idea and also making the use of helmets widespread. The College of Surgeons estimates that this measure has collectively saved many hundreds of Australian children from either serious brain damage or death.

Other states have since shown commendable initiatives to increase the use of helmets. Apart from the human tragedy of a maimed child, the community cost of medical treatment for a seriously brain-damaged child is put at $100,000 over five years. The bicycle helmet story shows what governments and concerned doctors and parents can do to create a safer environment for children.

Improvements, of course, still need to be made. A major misconception is that a sports helmet will give the participant absolute protection from head and neck injuries. The helmet just may not be strong enough to survive some severe impact. On the other hand, the helmet may be designed to remain unbroken — but not able to absorb the shock sufficiently to prevent injury to the wearer. Try to get a helmet which is one complete shell, rather than one with the two halves fused together.

Protective devices

Knee and elbow protectors, a proper visor or goggles (in races where there's a lot of dirt and mud), and wearing a good scarf like the promotorcyclists, can also be useful.

VISIBILITY FACTORS

Making sure a child can be seen should be a high priority. For night riding, don't forget to put a good light and reflectors on your child's bike. Again, it's all about paying attention to simple rules to avoid the risk of serious injury. Reflective tape is excellent — sew it onto the jacket or jumper a child likes wearing at night. The child should then be encouraged to carry this in his/her school bag, particularly in the winter months when even late afternoons mean poor visibility.

SAFETY HABITS

Wearing bicycle helmets should become as automatic as wearing seatbelts is. The more it becomes routine, the easier it is to do and the less conscious children become about doing it. Thanks to the campaigns by the Road Trauma Committee of the Royal Australasian College of Surgeons, Australians should be proud of having the highest record of seat belt-wearing in the world! It amazes people wherever we go that the first thing we do in getting into a car is to put the seat belt on. No matter if it's Yugoslavia, Britain, France or, particularly, the United States.

When I lived in the United States, my medical colleagues were amazed to see our children look for a seat belt when they got into a car and put it on before the car moved off. They were really surprised about how conditioned we had become about seat belts.

The most convincing argument to counter the question of infringement of civil liberty is the tremendous improvement in the morbidity of our road accident figures. I still get angry when I see parents driving with seat belts on but allowing their children to jump around in the back seat or lie unrestrained in the back of a station wagon! Those children become projectiles as soon as the driver has to brake hard. Unlike the car, which will decelerate from, say, 100 km/h, the unrestrained children in the back won't! The children will simply keep travelling at that speed. That's the speed at which they hit the windscreen.

I have seen children who have gone through the windscreen — in a hospital casualty department. The parents are often not injured but the child is dead. There are no words for such an easily preventable tragedy.

The key point here is that many, many more children are killed or seriously injured while riding in cars than while riding on BMX bikes, skateboards, rollerblades or horses. But we still need to train children to automatically put on a helmet when they go bike riding (or BMXing, or skateboarding or rollerblading or horse riding), just the way they put on seatbelts when they get into a car.

Making sure a child can be seen should be a high priority.

We still need to train children to automatically put on a helmet.

For skateboarders and rollerbladers, proper limb protection is especially important.

Good padding around handlebars and crossbars is important protection.

Teaching Children to Ride

The best accident prevention device isn't on sale in the shops. It's you! Parents should be involved in the learning phase. Make the time, because being there can make all the difference.

Busy streets

Far too many parents are still training their children on the street. Every year, the police accident statistics tell a grim story of the number of children with new bikes knocked down in January and February. So, stay off busy streets in the learning phase and stick to your backyard, driveway, a park with a bicycle track or the wide open expanses of an empty supermarket carpark. In fact, anywhere that's flat and where they can have a spill without the sudden crisis of a car zooming around the corner.

Confidence

Encourage them with training wheels and then raise the training wheels slowly, to allow them to develop more confidence. It's vital that they get your help and encouragement in that initial learning phase where they are particularly vulnerable to having a bad fall which will not only shake their confidence but also will often lead to a bad fracture when they instinctively put out a hand to cushion the fall.

Back to school

Always beware the first two weeks back at school. The number of children killed or seriously injured leaps between Christmas Day and the end of February. A multitude of children are still unsteady on the bicycles they got for Christmas and now want to ride to and from school. There are hundreds of near-misses in February with new school uniforms, strange shoes and new bikes. Combine this with a motorist running late for work and you have a prescription for disaster.

Get involved

It really pays tremendous dividends to get involved with your children. Even when you are doing the garden, it's a great idea to get one of your young children, who is learning to ride a bicycle, to join you. Parental involvement now will be an investment in your child's future, as well as being enjoyable at the time.

No matter how much you train your children on a bike, situations will still arise where a combination of factors will lead to a spill. If they have taken all the proper safety precautions, then serious injury risks are minimised. It's a big help if they practise falling off their bike onto grass. BMX track coaches can give excellent training in falling techniques, to minimise the risk of broken arms or collarbones.

If there's no BMX track, then try to form a parents' group and approach the local council to get one. If all else fails, there's always the local park. It's better than your son or daughter learning on the road where the 'tuition fees' could be high.

PREVENTING INJURIES

The most common injury to children who fall off BMX bikes, skateboards or horses is a fractured forearm or collarbone. Children are most vulnerable to falls when learning to ride. The single most important piece of prevention advice is for a parent to be there, to at least reduce the risk of a serious spill.

Protective equipment should be the other cornerstone of BMX riding, skateboarding and rollerblading.

GROIN INJURIES

Skeletal injuries and groin injuries are increasingly common as the popularity of BMXing spreads. Girls are not immune from injury. Sports medicine doctors are increasingly seeing bruising, and bleeding to the vulva (the external area around the vagina) with so many girls now engaging in BMX riding, and even just riding their brothers' BMX bikes, and hitting themselves between the legs with the crossbar. So it is important to get good padding around the handlebars and crossbars to protect the child's teeth and groin.

LIMB INJURIES

Proper limb protection is particularly important for skateboard riders because they are so prone to falling off when trying new jumps on ramps. A lot of the ramps are concrete and a heavy fall on concrete is very different from a fall onto a wooden surface. In skateboard riding, riders tend to land very heavily on their elbows and knees. This tends to mean bad bruising and possibly even damage to the elbow joint, the knee joint and the patella femoral joint.

The latter can get bruised and the cartilage of the lining on the joint can get badly damaged. Such injuries can happen in a second and can take months or years to get over. Skateboard riders should realise the tremendous stresses they are putting on their lower body, particularly below the knees, compared with their upper body, which is balanced and not stretched as much.

ANKLE INJURIES

Ankle sprains and irritations feature prominently on the casualty list for skateboard riders. They're particularly prone to Achilles tendon problems because of the frequency of leaning over and stretching their Achilles tendon and its supporting muscles up and down.

> **STOP**
> A proper SAA-approved helmet should always be worn.

Parents should be involved in the learning phase.

RIDING IN BMX CLUBS

Riding in BMX clubs is highly recommended. They're big on commonsense safety. Learning proper safety habits early on maximises injury-free enjoyment of the sport. Clubs are closely supervised. Well-padded handle bars are required before riders are allowed out on the track.

Another big plus is that the tracks don't have traffic hazards. Children are riding in an environment which is safe compared to roads full of unpredictable motorists involved in 'dodgem car' driving, negotiating trucks, roadworks and other hazards.

Children should develop their skills on BMX tracks by riding over jumps and moguls (little hills) and being taught how to land correctly. Such education in defensive riding is the best way to avoid injuries.

You need an experienced rider to teach the novice how to twist and turn and achieve the experts' tremendous aerial dexterity. Children have to learn in a low-risk situation. Then it's practice, practice, practice to perfect manoeuvres and stunts.

What is a piece of cake on a proper BMX track can be inviting disaster for a BMX daredevil on a suburban street. Streets are not playgrounds. Get kids into safe areas. Don't be complacent. Know where your kids are playing and know who they're playing with.

Keep children off busy streets.

MUSCLES

Skateboard riders' thighs and hamstrings come a close second in vulnerability and so should be included in the warm-up. This is a basic preventive measure which cannot be overstressed.

Any skateboard rider serious about the sport should always do a warm-up stretch lasting 10 to 15 minutes, particularly of their calves, the Achilles tendon and the muscles around their ankles just before a competition. Doing circles with the feet is highly recommended, as are toe and heel raises.

This warm-up advice applies particularly to skateboarding but also to BMX devotees.

HEAD INJURIES

You wouldn't whack a computer on a piece of concrete, and your brain is vastly more delicate than a computer, so treat it with the respect it deserves. A proper SAA-approved helmet should always be worn when riding, skateboarding or rollerblading. While not as good as a modern helmet, even an old-fashioned soft bicycle racing helmet is better than nothing.

With a head injury, we always talk about 'contra coup' injuries. This means that sometimes you can be hit on the back of the head but the front of the brain has been damaged, or vice versa. You have to remember that the brain is suspended in fluid inside the skull. It floats. Not a lot, but there's a little bit of give in there.

If you get hit from behind, the brain is sometimes pushed forward and hits the hard part at the front. It's easy to be misled about the neurological signs of the head injury. A person may be hit at the front and show signs of bruising of the brain at the back, so there can be bizarre signs when you're trying to work it out.

Treatment

The signs of a head injury are the same in any sport. If your child has fallen off a skateboard or a bike and hit his/her head, ask if he/she lost consciousness or remembers blacking out even for a moment. Always check what part of the head was hit. This information may be invaluable later. Ask if he/she has a headache, feels sick or has vomited. If you're unsure or unhappy with the situation, always err on the side of caution and take the child to the local hospital to be checked.

INTERNAL BLEEDING

A head injury may just be bruising of the brain. If it is very minor bruising, only be a headache. There may be some other signs but without long-term problems.

Really serious consequences arise from bleeding into the area where the brain is situated. Remember that the brain is sitting in a solid box. So any increase of fluid there, or any other thing which occupies space, for example, a tumour or bleeding, is going to cause increased pressure.

There are two types of bleeding: bleeding from an artery and bleeding from a vein. If it's arterial bleeding, the deterioration of the person's brain function will be very rapid because pressure is building up quickly from the heavy bleeding into the brain area. A person may collapse, feel nauseous, start vomiting and show pressure on their nerves such as the pupil of an eye dilating. The affected eye is usually on the opposite side of the brain from where the blood is collecting. The pupil may start getting bigger and bigger compared to the other side. If you see any of these signs, take the child straight to hospital. I would bypass the local doctor: he or she will only refer the child to hospital immediately. Such injuries need to be treated rapidly to avoid severe long-term consequences.

Treatment

Specialised tests such as X-rays and scans have to be taken immediately. Initial tests may show the person has a subarachnoid haemorrhage. In simple lay terms, this means serious arterial bleeding due to the bursting of an artery or a vessel. This doesn't necessarily mean there will be bleeding from an ear or ears. Bleeding from the ear or the nose is usually caused by a fracture at the base of the skull. Bleeding in the brain may not produce any obvious physical signs. There may only be a subtle neurological sign that no one

Really serious consequences can arise from head injuries.

> *The initial warning signs are dilating pupils, a very severe headache, double vision, or even collapse.*

except a doctor can detect.

Someone injured like this may feel fine immediately after the blow. They get up but then they can go off suddenly. When this happens, the deterioration is very rapid, within minutes. They may collapse, they may have problems breathing and they may need mouth-to-mouth resuscitation because of respiratory difficulties. That part of the brain which tells the lungs to work is malfunctioning. Remember, the initial warning signs are dilating pupils, a very severe headache, double vision, or even collapse. If you are concerned about any of these things, take the child straight to a medical centre. If the child has collapsed, there's nothing you can really do except put all sirens on and get the patient to the nearest hospital as quickly as possible. You need a major hospital with comprehensive facilities, such as the Royal Children's Hospital in Melbourne or the Royal Alexandria Hospital for Children in Sydney.

If the child is having breathing difficulties, you should apply mouth-to-mouth resuscitation. Fortunately, the respiratory centre isn't usually badly affected. This is the scenario of the fast deterioration — the most obvious one, where clearly something is seriously wrong.

The other, more subtle, scenario is delayed deterioration. Typically, the child comes home and says: 'I've bumped my head today, Mum.' You do a quick examination and can't see anything outwardly wrong. After a while, the headache subsides and the child says he/she feels all right. You relax and soon forget about it. The pressure on the brain may be building up very slowly and the deterioration is much more subtle. Then, somewhere about a week to two weeks later, your child starts to deteriorate without warning.

He or she may collapse, showing the signs of an acute bleed, even though it can be up to two weeks after the injury. The culprit is almost certainly a venous leak. This simply means a vein has been damaged.

Remember, during the two weeks after your child has had a knock to the head, be especially alert.

He or she may be having trouble concentrating at school, or may even suffer amnesia. If such symptoms occur, or you notice any other unusual behaviour, get the child to a doctor immediately. There are subtle signs indicating a venous bleed which you can look for before the child collapses and goes into that dangerous phase. Typical symptoms include some changes in the pupil and some changes in perception of light. This is because there are some nerves which deteriorate very quickly, particularly those to the eyes. The sixth cranial nerve is a nerve to the muscles of the eye which produces movement of the eyeball. It's one of the first nerves to be affected if you have some generalised pressure building up in the brain. Essentially, however, I'm

> *The other, more subtle, scenario is delayed deterioration.*

saying that it's wise to play safe.

If the child has had a head injury and if, over the next few days, he/she still feels a bit off or queasy, then get a medical examination.

The doctor will probably say, 'Because there's been a very significant blow to the head, I would like to see him/her again in the next few days.' This is not the doctor wanting to get another consultation fee. Rather, the doctor wants to check for signs of what we call a subdural haemorrhage.

This advice is for coaches as well as parents. Always err on the side of caution and get your child checked. Someone might wonder why a patient is kept for four hours in casualty with a head injury. The answer is that he/she is under observation for a subarachnial haemorrhage. This will usually show up within about four hours.

CONCUSSION

One of my pet hates in this society is the 'concussion scenario'. Australians take head injuries far too lightly. This attitude is at the elite level of players, administrators and the press (which moulds sporting heroes). Sports medicine practitioners are often dismayed about how this short-sighted, complacent attitude filters right down to the junior level.

The attitude is that if it's good enough for such and such a star player, then it's good enough for my son or daughter. It's a follow on from the public reaction to a brat tennis player abusing the umpire, for instance — the idea is then popularised for a lot of children and their parents.

Concussion is a closed head injury. (A closed injury is one where there's no cut and possibly no fracture.) Concussion is not usually a subarachnial nor a subdural injury. They are the big problems. But you still have bruising and damage to some part of the brain tissue. It may only be minor.

Treatment

My policy with any football team I have been the doctor for was that anyone had a serious head injury who had at least one of the following:

- sustained a concussion significant enough either to be taken from the ground or to have had difficulty walking off at the end of the game;
- felt sick and sometimes vomited;
- had a headache; and/or
- had suffered a transient loss of consciousness.

Sometimes the players used to try pulling the wool over my eyes because they knew my rule about anyone with a possible head injury not being allowed to play for two weeks. I am emphatic about this rule applying to kids. They should not return to BMX, skateboard riding, rollerblading, horse riding or any other position of risk, because *they are susceptible to even further damage* if they have another fall or another knock on the head.

Take a child to hospital if you are unsure about the injury.

Anyone with a possible head injury should not play for two weeks.

Be alert about any trouble a child has within two weeks of a head injury.

BOXING, HEAD INJURIES AND HELMETS

Without doubt, head injuries are the number one danger in all riding sports. Boxing is a perfect example of why you should protect your head from hard blows in any sport. Boxing is a sport where the brain is subjected to sharp blows. Look at the numerous brain-damaged boxers!

The human brain was simply not intended to take a series of severe shocks. That's what a hard impact is in a fall from a BMX bike, skateboard, rollerblades or a horse — and that's what boxing is, no more and no less. Every time your boy gets punched in the head, his brain will just bounce in the solid bone box which is the skull.

That's why padded helmets are so important (in a spill from a BMX bike, skateboard, rollerblades or a horse) compared to helmets with minimal padding. A well-padded helmet can greatly reduce brain damage.

Remember that the more the brain spins or bounces around on the spinal cord, the more chance there is of tearing arteries, rupturing veins and causing bleeding.

For these very good reasons, many doctors believe boxing is a definite 'no-no'. But as with any controversy, there's a counter-argument. In the final analysis, the simple advice is: think very carefully before you let your son or daughter take it up.

Don't overlook the fact that once a child has had a heavy spill, the material lining of his/her helmet may no longer have adequate shock-absorbing qualities. Crash helmets should be replaced after any major impact. This precautionary move is essential even if they don't appear damaged!

Taking unnecessary risks to save money can be a very expensive proposition if you're landed with a sports injury that will sideline you for months — or maybe permanently.

This is also why a helmet is one piece of gear you should never buy secondhand. It's virtually impossible to tell whether its previous owner has been involved in a mishap. Remember, helmets have practical limitations.

In the United States, where football tackling was practised with a helmet against a crush bag, mishaps were found to be unexpectedly prevalent. Often the crush bags were spring-loaded and thus accelerated against the oncoming tackle at considerable momentum. Any mistiming of the tackle meant that the neck could be hyperextended very easily or even flexed with dangerous consequences — despite the intact helmet.

A helmet is one piece of gear you should never buy secondhand.

This may sound tough, but many neurosurgeons would say this advice still doesn't go far enough. It's been shown that even if there's been only a very minor contusion to the brain, hand–eye coordination and other aspects of neurological function are still down, sometimes 6 to 12 months later. You are therefore at risk not only of a further head injury but also of another injury if you return to a sport requiring a high level of hand–eye coordination, particularly a contact sport.

How many times have you read in the sports pages that a player with severe concussion is bravely going to play next week? This is incredibly reckless behaviour. This is the coach and the administration dictating to the medical profession, trying to get their money's worth out of a player. Such a trivialisation of head injuries is playing Russian roulette. Sooner or later, the live round must come up in the firing chamber.

Sadly, Australia is not yet a truly professional football country, because we still do such stupid things. Take the example of the United States, where a pro footballer or baseball player can be worth $10 million. When I was studying specialised sports medicine in the United States, and was with pro football and baseball teams in the major leagues, it was brought home to me again and again that the players were too valuable to put at risk. The firm rule was that any player knocked unconscious didn't play for at least two weeks and usually three weeks. If they had a second serious head injury in the same year, then they didn't play for the rest of the year. Three serious head injuries in the same year, such as being knocked unconscious or bad concussion, and they usually never play football again.

The head injury message is just as important for parents as for football coaches and administrators. *Never, never* be blasé about your son or daughter getting a blow to the head — whatever sport they are playing, or even if they just fall off the bike in the driveway or backyard.

Always look for any abnormal behaviour weeks after the accident and, if in any doubt whatsoever, seek medical advice. A medical practitioner knows the subtle signs to look for. If this book achieves nothing else, I will be delighted if I have got across this head injury message loud and clear.

Horse-riding injury prevention

Helmets

Let's look quickly at girl horse riders who don't like wearing helmets. There's a simple way to avoid arguments. Don't give them any choice in the matter. 'No helmet, no riding!' End of conversation.

I prefer helmets without airholes. The minor discomfort of a helmet without airholes is better than the hazard of low hanging branches snagging one of the airholes and the rider being jerked off and ending up with a broken arm or broken leg or, at the worst, spinal damage.

In the final analysis, it comes back to authority and the individual. Parents and riding instructors have to be firm to be kind. A brain-damaged child on a respirator isn't a pretty sight. I have personally seen so many parents with guilt feelings about letting their child ride without a

> **STOP**
> If a child has collapsed, take him/her to hospital.

Never be blasé about a blow to the head.

> **STOP**
> Replace crash helmets after any major impact.

Horse riders should wear elbow and knee pads.

helmet, that it's not easily forgotten. Marriages often break up, with parents blaming one another. How do you put dimensions on such tragedy hitting a family? Wearing a helmet is such cheap protection. It should be nothing less than a firm condition of their mounting their horse.

PADS

Horse riders would also do well to wear elbow and knee pads. Elbow pads can even be worn under a shirt.

FAMILIARITY

If riding in a new area, check the ground for obstacles. This is nothing less than the professionals do. Equestrians who compete always carefully check out the course. The statistical equation is that the younger a rider is and the less experienced, the better the candidate he or she is for a serious injury. Riders have to learn to play the numbers game in reverse by minimising the risk situations, leaving only the purely accidental situations which no amount of thorough planning can foresee. The motto for every horse rider should be, 'expect the unexpected and keep your mind on the job'. The professionals make sure they know the course blind, so that if the horse suddenly shies at a jump and turns away to the left, they don't crash into a tree around a blind bend. One reason amateurs so often get into trouble is that they haven't carefully surveyed the course and worked out a gameplan for extricating themselves from trouble at difficult sections. Practically anything can spook a horse, with unpredictable consequences.

THE HORSE

Another reason for fairly inexperienced riders coming to grief is that they are on a strange horse which proves a little too high-spirited. Make sure you know you can handle your horse.

INJURIES

A fall off any horse means great risk of injury. Such injuries are usually bad bruises, contusions and fractures — particularly to upper extremities. The most serious are head injuries.

Fractures to the upper and lower limbs can occur in horse riding. Basically, the rider is falling from a height, usually on uneven ground, so there are a lot of problems. The injuries to horse riders are similar to those of BMX riders, rollerbladers and skateboard riders.

SNOW-SKIING INJURY PREVENTION

Having a high level of fitness is the biggest single factor identified by many studies on how to reduce the high level of injuries among novice skiers. A close second is having the right equipment, followed by going out with at least two other skiers and not taking foolhardy chances.

Be particularly careful first thing in

the morning. Are you and your children warmed up? Do you know where you're going? Are you all wearing adequate clothes? Have you checked the weather forecast? Have you let someone in the ski lodge know where you're going? Be aware of trees and check the position of pylons. It pays to carefully check the map before you go out. If there isn't one supplied, then ask for one.

Next, are all bindings correct? Have you checked that all the equipment is working before you go out? Don't forget ski goggles. The glare of the snow can be very treacherous.

Follow all directions on the mountain. If it says 'avalanche area', stay well clear. Always ski with a party unless you're a very experienced skier. In most situations, you should be on the mountain with people who know that you're there and know where you're going.

With more experienced skiers, injuries tend to occur either just before lunch or the last run of the day, when they're tired. So, if you're up on the mountain and you're tired and you decide to have just one more run — *don't*.

INJURIES

Foot and ankle problems are likely with ill-fitting boots, particularly with hired equipment. Fortunately, the standard of hired equipment has improved dramatically.

As boots are above the ankle, they protect the ankle and subtalar joint. So it's the knee joint which is most vulnerable because it can be severely stressed with all the twisting, turning and pivoting. This is particularly the case with novice skiers when they get their skis all twisted up and go rolling over down the slope. That's when a knee injury is most likely.

The other most common injury to novice skiers is the spiral fracture of the tibia. When their skis get caught in the snow, they pivot and rotate when the bindings don't release. They are then twisting against an immovable force. Snap! They spirally fracture their tibia.

Another serious risk is patella tendonitis. With frequent bending, the forces applied to the anterior aspect of the knee joint can cause inflammation of the patella tendon.

While lower extremity injuries are more prevalent in skiers, you can also get injuries in the upper extremities. For example, 'ski stock thumb' — a painful rupture of the ulna collateral ligament, which supports the joint at the base of the thumb. This can easily happen when the stock in your hand gets caught in the snow and you go forward.

Finally, a 'pro-tip' for beginners: always tie your ski jacket around you if the weather is hot. Apart from a sudden weather change, you may get caught in a snow drift and you might be exposed overnight.

> *Always ski with a party unless you're a very experienced skier.*

ICE-SKATING INJURY PREVENTION

Injury prevention starts with a good stretching program and keeping up a good general level of fitness.

Ice skating always becomes high profile in the media when the winter Olympics are on. Children want to do it because of its grace and beauty.

Injury prevention starts with a good stretching program and keeping up a good general level of fitness with exercise. Flexibility has to be very good for a combination of endurance, speed and strength.

The most basic mistake is choosing poorly-fitting boots, which can cause blisters and other foot problems. Also, rolling over can cause some ankle injuries, even though you are wearing high-cut boots.

Knee and ankle pads are not usually worn but they are worth considering with the novice skater. Because of the gliding movements, falling on the elbows and knees doesn't cause as many problems here as with skateboarding, rollerblading and BMX riding. Novice ice skaters tend to land on their hips or bottoms. They can get contusions and bruises but these are usually minimal and the standard treatment of ice gives quick relief.

For the inexperienced, a lesson is a good idea or at least going with someone who knows what to do. If the novice is falling over a lot, then use an area that's safe, where there's not a lot of fast skating going on, so they don't get run into and end up with a serious injury or a serious laceration. You can even lose a finger if you fall with instinctively outstretched hands.

You should make sure that children and other novices are well supervised by a responsible adult.

Novice ice skaters should stay in the designated area so they can find their feet and balance before venturing out in the general area.

INJURIES

With more experienced skaters, it's common to see injuries similar to skateboarding and BMXing where there are also a lot of difficult twists and landings with heavy bruising to the elbows, knees and hips. Twisting injuries and muscle sprains occur because skaters put a lot of stress on their lower extremities with all the twisting and turning. They are similar to injuries in many other sports and the treatment is the same.

HELPFUL HINTS

- Know the track or course.
- Know how to land correctly from a fall.
- Wear correctly-fitting helmets and other appropriate protective equipment, such as elbow and knee protectors.
- Never take head injuries lightly. Always seek medical advice if unsure. Don't let a child return to sport for two to three weeks if he/she has been knocked out, or has had headaches or nausea after the head injury.
- With skiing, check the weather forecast, check that the boots and other equipment are suitable for the age group, and have suitable clothing in case the weather changes. Let someone know which area you are going to and what time you expect to be back. For safety's sake, ski in groups.

CHAPTER 8

RACQUET SPORTS: TENNIS, SQUASH AND BADMINTON

PREVENTIVE MEASURES

The most important preventive measure in racquet sports is the use of proper footwear. Since the boom of running sports, racquet sports have been largely neglected in this area. It's only been in the last five years that the sporting companies have developed really excellent sports shoes.

Shoes are very important because racquet sports involve twisting and turning in a confined area. Ankle injuries are common. Girls, particularly, have a high injury rate because they play such a lot of tennis, usually wearing inadequate shoes. There was an epidemic in 1982 of chronic ankle instability in young girl tennis players. Sports physicians found their patients had often been wearing very sloppy, loose-fitting or inadequate shoes.

It really wasn't until netball took off in Australia that people became more conscious of wearing the right type of shoes to reduce the chance of injury. Shoes became more fashionable. Reebok and other brands became more colourful and thus more appealing to wear.

The right footwear is also important when doing aerobics, but it is young adolescents rather than young children who have got into this in a big way.

ANKLE INJURIES

Unlike adults, children recover quickly from injury and may not need to see a doctor. Often, children do not even tell their parents that they have twisted their ankle. Their tissues are young, they're flexible and they're fit and although they have ankle pain with some swelling, they can return to activities very quickly. If they become a little concerned, they might report this to their mother or father and then the problem settles down with some ice treatment and a few days' rest. But in many cases they don't do the proper rehabilitation.

A sprained ankle is an acute injury which damages the ligaments of the ankle. The range can go from mild ligament damage to serious damage to muscles, tendons and bone.

A sprain occurs after a sudden movement that exceeds the range of motion of the ankle

A sprained ankle is an acute injury which damages the ligaments of the ankle.

joint. Without proper use, the problem can become chronic. Otherwise, the ankle should heal well and allow a safe, early return to activity.

The ankle joint consists of the tibia (shin bone), the fibula, the talus and the calcaneus. Inside the ankle, the joint is stabilised by the strong fibrous deltoid ligament. Sprains to this ligament ('eversion sprains') account for less than 20 per cent of ankle sprains.

Outside the ankle, the joint is stabilised by three ligaments, the anterior talofibular (at the front), the calcaneofibular (at the side) and the posterior talofibular (at the back).

More than 80 per cent of all ankle sprains are to the outside of the foot, as the range of movement for inversion (turning of the foot) is greater than for eversion. This is due to the anatomy of the foot.

LACK OF EXERCISE

The most serious omission, which condemns most athletes to reinjury, is that they don't do an exercise program to strengthen the injured area. Furthermore, if they return too quickly, they might just get little recurrent sprains of the lateral ligaments of the ankle and the subtalar joint, the joint just below the ankle joint. This often proves to be the last straw on the camel's back, and the muscles get continually weaker to the point of failure.

About the most common ankle sprain, which I have referred to in other chapters, is the inversion injury of the foot. The foot turns in and there is damage to the outer or lateral ligament. During an examination of this injury, you typically find the ligaments are a little lax. Possibly the most important finding is that the muscles are significantly weaker compared with the other side when you do a subjective resistance test of the muscle supporting the joint.

Testing for the strength of muscles is now much easier with specialised machines. The first was a Cybex, and now there are several other excellent ones on the market which can accurately evaluate the strength of a muscle. These machines are able to test the muscles either isotonically or isometrically, and then exercise them isokinetically. The isokinetic aspect of a muscle is its strength measured against an accommodating force.

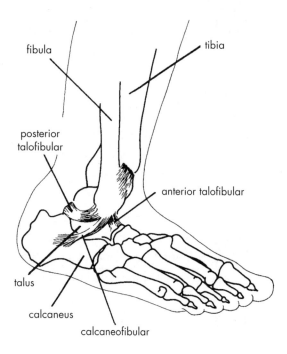

Isometric muscle strength is when you are testing the strength of a muscle against an immovable force. For example, when you are applying force through a muscle in leaning against a wall.

Isotonic muscle strength is the strength of a muscle as it's moving a weight against a variable resistance. As the weight is lifted higher against gravity, the resistance becomes greater.

The big advantage of the machines is that they give a graphic read-out and allocate an actual value to the strength of these muscles of the knee, hip, shoulder, wrist, elbow and ankle. Thus, these machines have become increasingly important in precisely assessing the level of muscle weakness.

There's also a machine for lower back assessment. This has been a boon for physiotherapists and orthopaedic physicians and surgeons in improving testing and simple rehabilitation programs for the relief of chronic muscle instability. But these wonderful advances should not obscure the fact that prevention of thousands of such injuries a year is the best policy of all!

Prevention of ankle injuries comes down to two things:

- wear good shoes; and
- no matter how minor an ankle sprain, have it looked at and given a proper exercise program. For a child, this usually means a week for the problem to clear up.

In the early phases, a range of movement is important. Apply a resistance exercise program to avoid stiffness in the joint, particularly the ankle.

The problem of chronic ankle instability shouldn't exist in children and young adolescents if you follow this simple rule: if a child gets an ankle sprain, treat it correctly, quickly and efficiently.

If you suspect that a child has a tendency to fall over, or has any other problem with an ankle, have the child checked. An exercise program is also advised to strengthen their forehand before they start playing tennis.

WARM-UPS ARE ESSENTIAL

A warm-up is essential in all racquet sports. It's very simple to just go onto the court, start playing and doing a 'hit up'. That's not the proper warm-up needed to avoid injury. Proper exercises have to be done to adequately prepare muscles and joints.

In tennis, squash and badminton, the vital areas to work on are the tendo-Achilles, the shoulder and upper limb muscles. In particular, the elbows and wrists should be flexible enough to give them a range of movement up and down. In general, get the muscles working.

Elbows and shoulders should be worked through the full range of movement. Forwards, moving from the side, extending slowly, and then stretching the quads and the hamstrings of the thigh muscles. See Stretching Exercises, page 9.

The most basic mistake is choosing poorly fitting shoes.

You should always have an exercise program to strengthen the injured area.

ANKLE SPRAINS

CAUSE

1 Previous injury
2 Compensation for other injury
3 Inappropriate/worn out shoes
4 Uneven surface

TREATMENT

1 Immediate: ICE
   Ice (crushed ice in a damp towel)
   Compression (tensor bandage)
   Elevation (using pillows, elevate above level of heart)

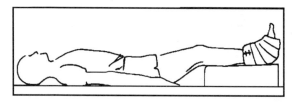

Above: Ice compression and elevation.

Ice should be applied within minutes of the injury. The sooner it is applied, the less the secondary damage will be, with more effective rehabilitation and faster recovery. Leave ice in position for 20 to 30 minutes. Then remove ice and re-apply compression and elevation. Continue compression and elevation constantly for one to three days, depending on the severity of the injury. Apply ice every two hours, for 20 to 30 minutes.

Right: Making an ice pack.

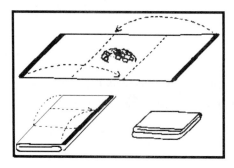

2 Anti-inflammatory medication may be prescribed.

3 Begin mobilisation immediately, through movements within a pain-free range of motion.

4 Crutches should be used if the person is unable to walk normally without pain or a limp.

5 Physiotherapy can help to achieve a full recovery, through a combination of ice and exercise.

EXERCISE

Start mobilisation exercises immediately to prevent scarring and to restructure a strong ligament. Exercises may be uncomfortable but should not be painful. One set of exercises leads to the next.

1 Range of motion (ROM) exercises — circles, up and down, in and out, alphabet with big toes.
When range of motion in the injured ankle is equal to the uninjured, strength exercises are started. ROM exercises should be continued.

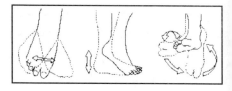

Above: ROM exercises, in and out, up and down, circles.

2 Tube and towel exercises — three sets of ten for each exercise. As this gets easier, it can be made harder by increasing tension on the tube or putting weights or books on the end of the towel.

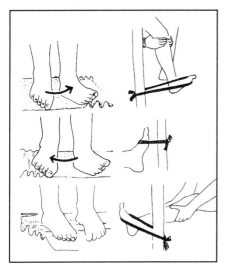

Above: Tube and towel exercises.

RETURN TO ACTIVITY

Some protection is needed for the ankle for at least six months, as remodelling of the ligament is not complete until then. Taping is the best, and supports or braces are an option. High-cut sports shoes should be worn.

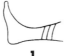

1   Anchors.

2   Three stirrups (start on inside leg, down, under foot and up on outside leg).

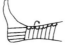

3   Closing anchors.

4   Heel lock.

3 When able to stand pain-free, begin proprioception exercises. Begin by standing on the injured foot for three seconds and gradually work up to '747s' (30 seconds each, repeat entire sequence three times).
This progression may take from one week to three to four months.
When able to hop ten times and stand on toes of injured ankle for 20 seconds, progress to next step and continue 747s daily.

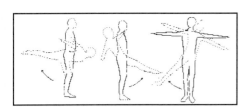

Above: 747s.

4 Jogging in straight line, gradually progressing to 'S' jogging or large '8s', and eventually to cuts, zigzags, stop and starts. When the zigzags can be done pain-free without support, athlete can return to sport and activity.

Tube and towel exercises and proprioception exercises should be continued on a daily basis, although they should be done after a practice or game, not before.

Racquet Sports 95

PATHOLOGY OF ANKLE SPRAINS

DEGREE OF INJURY	EXTENT	TREATMENT	PROGNOSIS
First-degree (mild)	Mild tearing and stretching of ligaments	Immediate ice, compression, elevation for 1 to 2 days	Return to sport 3 days to 2 to 3 weeks
	Mild swelling, if any	Strengthen muscles	
	No instability	Balance exercises	
Second-degree (moderate)	Partially-torn ligaments	Immediate ice, compression, elevation for 2 to 3 days	3 to 6 weeks before return to full activities
	Involves injury to 1 or more of the ligaments	Crutches or cane	
	Swelling and bruising	Physiotherapy	
Third-degree (severe)	Complete rupture of 2 or more ligaments	Immediate ice, compression, and elevation, continue for 2 to 3 days	Can be 8 to 12 months for ligaments to fully heal
	May involve a fracture	X-ray	
	Swelling, bruising	After 3 days continue compression during day.	
	Pain on opposite side of sprain due to compression of tissue and bone	Physiotherapy. Surgery rarely required	

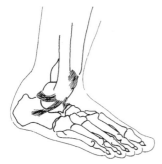

First-degree (mild)

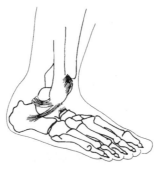

Second-degree (moderate)

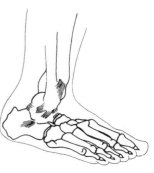

Third-degree (severe)

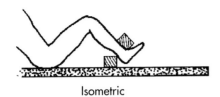
Isometric

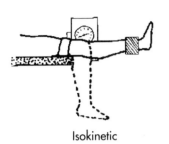
Isokinetic

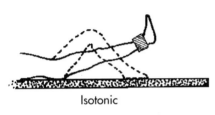
Isotonic

Strengthening exercises for the hamstring and quadriceps muscles. These show the three modes of exercise for muscle strengthening.

AVULSION INJURIES

Racquet sports are notorious for tendo-Achilles problems — either a partial or complete rupture. Mainly adults suffer this because they're playing vigorously. Children tend to be more flexible. They get more of an irritation of their tendo-Achilles. The other important point with the younger players is that tendons, particularly near the attachment to bone, are stronger.

The consequence for children is a greater chance of an avulsion of a ligament or tendon around a joint. An avulsion is when a ligament or a tendon, instead of rupturing when the force is applied, tends to pull off where it's attached to the bone. This is because a tendon or ligament is usually stronger than the bone in the area where the tendon is attached.

Such avulsion injuries in the tendo-Achilles or in ligaments around the knee and elbow are common in children.

Treatment

An avulsion can take two to six months to heal. In general, it's not necessary to operate on an avulsion injury. The best treatment is RICE, rest and protection, a carefully increasing rehabilitation program and a cautious return to sporting activity.

HEEL INJURIES

In young males between 11 and 14 years, it's common to see Sever's Disease with the secondary growth plate on the heel bone becoming irritated or inflamed.

Children with this condition don't always stop playing, because they're so resilient. The problem just builds up. When the discomfort gets too much to put up with, they tell their parents, who seek medical help. The doctor invariably finds either a history of running long distances, or that they've been on a long hike or have been playing a lot of tennis, squash or netball on a hard surface.

These injuries to the heel are usually jarring injuries. Children get pain and a gradual limp. The pain is aggravated by low heels, standing on

Treat an ankle sprain correctly, quickly and efficiently.

Injuries to the heel are usually jarring injuries. Children get pain and a gradual limp.

A rupture of the tendo-Achilles can be missed by young players and sometimes even by their doctors.

Racquet sports are notorious for tendo-Achilles problems.

A CAUTIONARY TALE

The following cautionary tale applies equally to children and to adult squash players. I was a young doctor on night duty in a casualty department of a large public hospital in Melbourne when two injured squash players came in. They were good mates but had become pretty intense about their squash. One presented in casualty with a black eye and a broken nose. The other was badly bruised about the face.

I was curious about why they had such a bad fight on the squash court. As I was patching one of them up for a broken knuckle I got the blow-by-blow description of how they had hit the walls as they fought and rolled around. He said, 'I really don't know why it happened. My mate suddenly went crazy and started thumping me!'

So I went into the next cubicle and started to treat his companion's head injuries. He was in a fair amount of pain and he started moaning and groaning. 'Why did you start it?' I asked him.

'My right leg was killing me around the calf area. That's what happened. I was playing a shot and he was behind me and he kicked or hit me with his racquet right at the back of my leg. I was in agony so I turned around and thought that, because I was beating him, he was getting narky and had decided to have a go at me.'

When I examined his leg I found that he had completely ruptured his tendo-Achilles. When that happens, it can be like a pistol shot, the pain is so intense. Anyone in this situation could be excused for thinking that their opponent had either kicked them hard in the back of the leg or whacked them with a racquet. This rather innocent on-court injury led to them both ending up in casualty. But the most serious injury of all remained the ruptured tendo-Achilles!

This misunderstanding and instant suspicion of your opponent, even in a friendly game of squash, is more common than most players realise.

A total rupture of the tendo-Achilles needs to be sutured fairly quickly. This injury can be missed by young players and sometimes even by their doctors. The classic test is to lie them on their stomach with their feet hanging over the edge of the bed. A doctor only has to run his or her finger down to find the problem because the tendo-Achilles is such a lovely, firm tendon that the break is very definite.

tip toes and pressure on the back of heels. Usually the doctor does an X-ray and this might show some changes in the growth plate. It may also be necessary to do a nuclear bone scan and a CT scan (computerised tomography). The symptoms are usually short-lived and recurrences are common until the growth plate has finished growing.

Treatment

The treatment is to relieve the tension on the growth plate and this means using a heel pad to elevate the heel a little. Alternatively, strap the foot to hold it in a position where the heel is raised to take the pressure off the growth plate. As mentioned earlier, this can be a common thing in boys 11 to 14. So, when they present with heel pain, the doctor should suspect Sever's Disease, or a tendo-Achilles inflammation.

UPPER LIMB INJURIES

Injuries to the upper limbs are a significant problem with players of racquet sports. The major ones are shoulder injuries, especially rotator cuff irritation. The rotator cuff is the common group of tendons of muscles which produce the rotatory movements of the arm at the shoulder joint. Inflammation of one or several of these muscles, particularly in the tendons, can cause pain when the arm is being moved up or from the side and rotating it (for example, serving in tennis).

This injury occurs mainly because of overuse when playing a lot of tennis. In tennis, players tend to hit from the elbow with the wrist firm. They use more of their elbow and shoulder. So it's probably more common in tennis and badminton, which also involve a lot of overhead movements.

It's less common in squash because there are fewer overhead movements. Squash is a more wristy sport than tennis. Players tend to hit vigorously from the side. If they are playing good squash, then the wrists and forearms can take a surprising amount of punishment without the player realising it. In squash, therefore, inflammation of the capsule and ligaments in the wrist can occur.

Treatment

Again, the treatment is rest, ice and maybe taking some anti-inflammatory medication.

If a shoulder injury persists, it may be worthwhile contemplating some long-acting local anaesthetic or a cortisone injection into the bursa (the sac which is bathing the area with fluid around the common tendon group). This is a very effective way of getting an anti-inflammatory into that area.

Cortisone injections, if used correctly, are usually very effective, provided they go into a space bathing a tendon and not into a tendon or a muscle itself. Cortisone is a very effective anti-inflammatory. It works by reducing the tissue's natural inflammatory response. This in turn allows the tissues to heal and recover. So if it's injected directly into a tendon, the area becomes very weak and can eventually rupture.

It's wise to consult a sports medicine specialist if your GP hasn't had a lot of experience with a resistant tennis elbow or rotator cuff inflammation, particularly in treating a young adolescent, or if the condition hasn't resolved itself with normal treatment methods or physiotherapy.

Cortisone works by reducing the tissue's natural inflammatory response.

TENNIS ELBOW AND ELBOW PAIN

Tennis elbow is caused by the forces generated by the backhand.

A proper warm-up is the preventive measure for tennis elbow.

Tennis elbow is a significant problem with young tennis players although probably not as prevalent as it is with adults. Tennis elbow is classically the description of pain over the outer, or lateral, aspect of the elbow joint. It gained its name because it is very common in tennis players. It is caused by the forces generated by the backhand. Backhand movements require extension of the wrist or firmness of the extensor muscles. The lateral aspect of the elbow joint is the origin of the extensor muscles to the wrist. Thus, a traction injury can occur when applying a very strong force to this area. This can cause inflammation of the actual bone and tenosynovitis of the muscle origin. Inflammation of a small joint

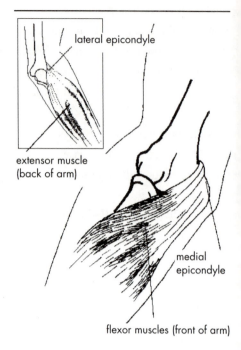

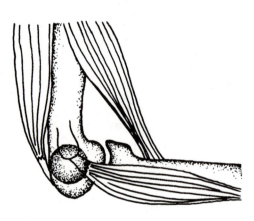

Tennis elbow is commonly a combination of inflammation of the outer aspect of the elbow joint, especially involving the origin of the extensor muscles.

between the humerus bone of the upper arm and the radius, a forearm bone, can also cause pain and restrict movements of the elbow and forearm. A proper warm-up is the preventive measure for tennis elbow.

There are three bumps in the elbow. The largest is not important in tennis elbow — it involves the two less distinct bumps, on the inside (the 'medical epicondyle'), and on the outside (the 'lateral epicondyle'). Hence the medical terms, 'lateral epicondylitis' to describe pain on the outside bump and 'medial epicondylitis' to describe pain on the inside bump. Pain may also occur in the muscles attached to these bumps.

Causes

Injury occurs gradually as small injuries occur repeatedly to the same area. These small injuries may result from unaccustomed use, improper technique, unsuitable equipment, lack of strength in the forearm muscles, or lack of flexibility in the wrist and elbow.

These small injuries may go unnoticed or only give minor discomfort, but over time they cause gradual damage where the muscle attaches to the bone. This is when the symptoms of the injury may occur.

Symptoms

These include pain on straightening the elbow, pain when attempting to curl fingers and/or wrist (for medial epicondylitis) or straighten fingers or cock wrist (for lateral epicondylitis), point tenderness and pain when lifting or grasping an object.

Immediate care

If the problem is minor, apply ice in the following ways:

- Ice massage: fill a paper cup with water. Freeze overnight. Remove the paper from the ice and gently rub over the bone and muscle for 15 minutes.
- Ice packs: wrap crushed ice in a damp towel. Wrap around the elbow with an elastic non-adhesive bandage. Leave for 15 to 20 minutes.
- Ice immersion for 15 to 20 minutes.

Treatment

The aim is to reduce inflammation, aid complete healing, and prevent recurrence by identifying and correcting the cause of the injury. Treatment may include an anti-inflammatory medication, as prescribed by your doctor. Your doctor may also suggest going to a physiotherapist. This is very important as it will assist complete healing of the injury and help prevent a recurrence.

Treatment may include:

- Ice and exercise
- Heat treatments
- Ultrasound
- Electrical muscle stimulation
- Combination of ultrasound and muscle stimulation
- Strength and flexibility exercises.

Injury prevention

- Stretch and strengthen, using the above exercies daily for two to three weeks before participating in the sport.

If the problem is minor, apply ice.

Your doctor may suggest going to a physiotherapist.

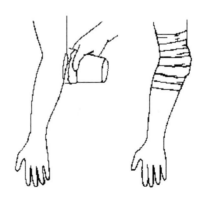
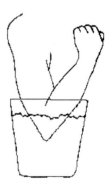

Ice massage, ice pack, ice immersion.

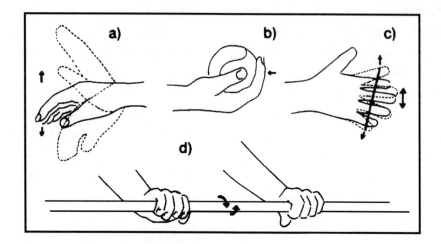

STRENGTHENING EXERCISES

1 Bending and straightening wrist
2 Squeezing a tennis ball
3 Finger exercises
4 Broom handle exercises.

FLEXIBILITY EXERCISES

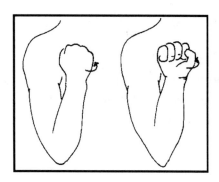

Left: Elbow flexion, fist pushed towards chest, back of fist pushed towards chest.
Below: Wrist flexions, extensions and flexions with bent fingers, finger abductions.

Three sets of ten for each exercise: hold each one for 6 to 10 seconds. Gently and slowly stretch to the point of discomfort, not pain. Do at least once daily.

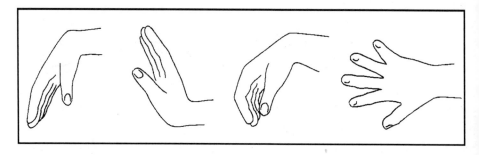

- Warm-up (include stretching) and warm-down (include stretching) after every practice, game or playing time.
- Use equipment appropriate for you.
- Concentrate on proper technique and/or modify your previous technique.
- Ice immediately at the first sign of problems, then seek advice.

Braces

Sometimes a brace worn around the forearm is effective in treating epicondylitis. The brace, or stretchy tape, is applied around the widest part of your forearm and worn during the activity (tennis, golf, etc) that originally caused the pain.

Normally, the brace should be worn for progressively less time until it need not be worn at all. Successful physiotherapy and practice of preventive measures should make the use of a brace needless.

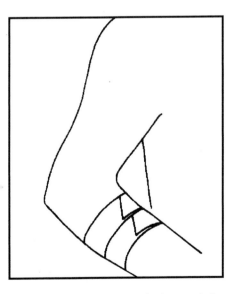

Brace, or stretchy tape, applied around the widest part of forearm.

Racquets

One of the most overlooked preventive measures is the type of racquet used. A child should never use a racquet with the wrong grip size. It's been found that the way a player grips the racquet has a great effect on the tension of the muscles in the forearm.

When medial epicondylitis is the problem, it's not the weight of the racquet which is critical here, it's the size of the grip. The important thing is to make sure that when you're buying a racquet, price isn't the only criterion.

It's important to buy from a place where they measure the child's hand to make sure the grip size and weight is right. It's also vital that the racquet should not be of a design that's inherently heavy. To measure for grip size, take a tape and measure from the tip of the middle finger to the mid-point of the palm of the hand. That distance is the size of the grip required.

There was a rapid increase in the prevalence of tennis elbow when a larger, oversize racquet head became popular and the average tennis player rushed to get it. With some of the racquets with oversized heads, the weight ratio from the head of the racquet down to the grip wasn't quite right. A lot of players were getting tennis elbow because of the imbalance. Always check for any warning signs of inflammation around the joint, because an early presentation of tennis elbow can be treated very effectively with proper management and exercises.

Rotator cuff irritation is common in tennis and badminton.

Wrist injuries are common in squash.

A proper warm-up is the best method of injury prevention.

EXERCISES FOR TENNIS ELBOW

There are three exercises which are basic for minimising the effects of tennis elbow and should be used by people who have had problems. Firstly, put the forearm flat on the desk or the table and do a hand clench with your wrist. Then bend your wrist down and back, up and down, up and down. Do at least 20 of these.

Secondly, put your elbow, bent, onto your head and do straightening and bending, working on your triceps muscle on the back of the upper arm.

Thirdly, I think the best exercise is one we devised at the Malvern Sports Medicine Clinic in Melbourne. We used to call it the 'Tennis Elbow Stretch'. It involves putting the back of your hands together, just as if you are going to do a breast stroke.

Keep the back of your wrists together and pull your hands back, keeping them straight. You can feel the tension of the muscle there as you go out. Hold this position for a count of 10 and then just relax. Do 20 of these.

I think such an exercise is important for anyone in the early stages of the treatment. So is the use of frictional massage, ice massage and possibly an anti-inflammatory.

You can do a combination of frictional and ice massage: by applying the ice you are doing a form of frictional massage. Also, do some friction with your fingers by simply rubbing over the area where the tendon, or the origin of the muscle, is on this bony part of your elbow.

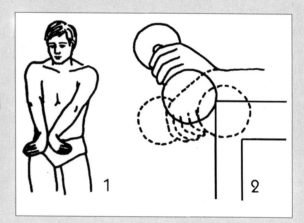

1 Tennis elbow stretching exercise for both elbows. The elbows and the hands are kept straight. The hands bend out at the wrists. Keep the back of the wrists together until pain is felt at the outer elbow region.

2 Strengthening exercise for the forearm extensor muscles using either a dumbbell or a convenient weight such as a sock filled with sand and weighing about 5 kilograms.

EYE INJURIES

A squash ball can move up to 190 km/h, and is smaller than the eye socket.

Eye injuries are common in squash and badminton. Any sport where a missile is smaller than the eye socket deserves commonsense precautions. You can be hit by a tennis ball and it can really irritate your eye but the ball is bigger than the bony socket. So it can cause some damage but the small risk makes it unnecessary to wear goggles.

The really big danger is the squash ball which can move at up to 190 km/h, and has a big potential for massive eye injuries because it is smaller than the eye socket. It can therefore hit the eyeball directly without any reduction in its velocity.

The eye sits in a bony box and, if you apply a rapid increase in the force within that bony box, something has to give. Either the eye will rupture, or one of the walls will rupture, and it's usually the floor. Known as a 'blow out' fracture, the eye can squeeze down through the floor of the orbit.

The result is a sunken eye as well as significant damage to the nerves of the eye, particularly the optic nerve of the eyeball. This can be permanent and may even cause blindness if the optic nerve has been severely damaged.

I see this as a potential danger across the whole age range. But while children playing squash are not going to hit the ball as fast as adults, it's an excellent idea to start them wearing goggles. When they go to play squash, they put on shoes, sweat band and eye goggles. Wearing them should become such second nature that they feel odd without them.

The danger is compounded by squash being in such an enclosed space that the ball can come at a player from really odd directions. It can bounce off any of the four walls as well as the floor. Thus it's mandatory in squash that you wear proper protective goggles at all times, no matter what age group you are in.

In tennis, there is a much greater chance of avoiding the ball because there is usually time to take evasive action unless, of course, the ball is smashed straight at the player.

In badminton, protective eye gear is a good idea but isn't as essential. The shuttlecock certainly doesn't go as fast as a squash ball. The feathers show it down. But in top grade badminton, you do occasionally see the players wearing goggles because the end of the shuttlecock is smaller than the eye socket.

It's mandatory in squash that you wear proper protective goggles at all times, no matter what age group you are in.

HELPFUL HINTS

- Injuries commonly involve the upper extremities (the shoulder, elbow and wrist) as well as the lower leg (especially tendo-Achilles inflammation).
- Always allow enough time for a good stretching warm-up.
- Match the racquet to the child.
- Grip size should match the size of the hand.
- With small ball sports such as squash and racquet ball, always wear protective eye glasses.
- Remember the size of the racquet head:
    a normal size head for juniors
    a mid-size head for adolescents and young adults
    veterans usually play with oversize racquets.

CHAPTER 9

NETBALL AND BASKETBALL

Basketball and netball are two big success stories of the sports scene in many countries. The National Basketball League is going from strength to strength, with aggressive recruiting campaigns in schools boosting the numbers of players every year. Netball is probably the most widely-played sport by women. Australia is the number one nation in the world in netball, with an estimated 750,000 women and girls playing it.

In such fast-moving and exhilarating games, injuries are inevitable. However, the treating of these sports injuries is often inadequate. This particularly applies to netball. Many injuries, if not most, go untreated. A tremendous improvement is needed. There should be absolutely no compromise — all injuries, minor as well as serious, need prompt attention.

I remember a late afternoon I spent at Melbourne's Royal Park. A sports trainer friend had asked me to go along to a mid-week match because he was concerned they didn't have any sports medicine advice. I thought I would volunteer an hour of my time because there would only be a few teams playing. Instead, I was amazed at the hundreds of girls in action! It was one of the major regional areas that play netball every night of the week. There were numerous games going on simultaneously, playing constantly and rotating around. The vigour, zest and enthusiasm were infectious.

I set up a mini-clinic there with my sports trainer friend. Within an hour, we had looked at eight girls who had sustained major knee injuries over the past few days. Then, in that first hour, there were six new injuries! They were the common injuries I talk about in this chapter — injuries to ankles, knees and fingers.

INJURY PREVENTION

Any large regional netball or basketball centre should have a physiotherapist or sports trainer on hand.

In view of the sheer numbers of netballers and basketballers, it's a tremendous service to have a trained person present to provide first aid treatment and to know when to refer a more serious injury to an appropriate sports medicine doctor, or a medical specialist if it's a really tricky injury.

Efforts have been made to deal with the lack of qualified personnel. There are now many good sports trainers at level 1 and level 2 as set by the Australian Sports Trainers Association, together with the Australian Sports Medicine Federation. Both organisations are to be commended for their efforts to improve sports injury prevention and treatment.

PARENTAL INVOLVEMENT

If your children play these sports, you, as a parent, can become involved and help improve the existing inadequate situation. As many parents as possible should learn basic first aid. Parents who attend games regularly should make sure there's a roster of people who have a first aid certificate. At every game, there should be someone available who can not only administer first aid but also recognise a more serious injury that needs the attention of a doctor or hospital.

Every parent and club official should know how to use RICE — rest, ice, compression, elevation — and also know that heat should never be applied to an injury. All heat does is promote bleeding and cause complications.

THE COURT

Basketball and netball are played on regular-sized courts which can be surveyed fairly quickly. It's important that the boundaries of the court are well marked and not close to fixed objects which players can run into.

Many basketball courts are squeezed into a small hall with little room between the side line and the wall. Consequently, players concentrating on watching the ball can run slap bang into the wall, causing themselves considerable injuries. At the very least, remove large objects such as tables and chairs.

Sweat is the hazard in all sports played on floors, particularly basketball. A surprising amount of sweat and moisture is generated in a game. A 'sweaty' floor can easily cause a slip, resulting in a significant injury to the back or a twisted ankle or knee. So always make sure that the court is wiped down before, during and after the game when playing on a polished floor.

Both basketball and netball can be played indoors or outdoors. When outdoors, they unfortunately tend to be played on asphalt, which can be mighty rough stuff. It can be hard on the feet, particularly on a hot day. Falling can mean a graze and an infection. You must be careful to get any wound cleaned thoroughly.

PROTECTIVE PADS

I don't think it's overly cautious to have children wearing BMX-style elbow and knee protection pads. With volleyball, the same principles apply.

You see more and more top-level basketballers wearing protective kneepads. Landing on the knee can damage the lining of the joint surface. The cartilage on the undersurface of the kneecap can be cracked and cause irritation and other problems. This happens in netball, basketball and volleyball.

SHOES

In basketball, netball and volleyball, there's a tendency to get ankle injuries with so much twisting and rolling over on the foot. Girls playing these sports should consider wearing

At every game, there should be someone available who can not only administer first aid but also recognise a more serious injury that needs the attention of a doctor or hospital.

A sweaty floor is dangerous, so make sure the court is constantly being wiped down.

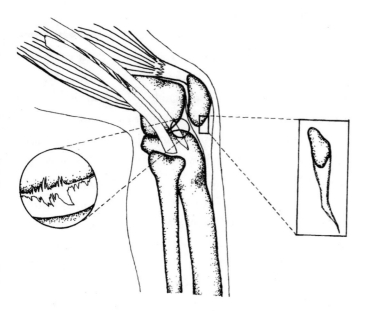

Anterior knee pain. There are many causes, usually patella tendon inflammation or articular cartilage damage.

Some people believe wearing high-cut shoes — that is, above the ankle joint — puts more stress on the knee joint.

I disagree because stresses on the knee joint are different from those on the ankle and cause totally different injuries. I believe that protecting your ankle by strapping or using high-cut boots doesn't make you any more vulnerable to knee injuries.

KNEE INJURIES

In netball, the knees are placed under tremendous stress when the player has to catch the ball, stop quickly and perhaps pivot. It's these movements which can damage the internal structures of the knee: the meniscus (the cartilage) and the cruciate and collateral ligaments.

Knee injuries are also common in basketball. The twisting, turning and sudden stopping, and the jumping and landing, can put stress on the knee joint. The anterior aspect of the knee, the patella tendon, can become inflamed above and below the kneecap and the patella femoral joint can become irritated.

The knee is always an area to watch.

Treatment

See Chapters 2 and 3 for a full discussion of the on-the-spot knee injury treatments. Long-term treatment again means looking at the factors which predispose children to such injuries. The injured child could have what is commonly called

higher-cut shoes to protect their ankles. The time-honoured shoe in these sports has been a low-cut black shoe made by Dunlop. However, there are now a greater variety of shoes being worn. While most are low cut for reasons of speed, children can still get a pair of high-cut shoes to provide that all-important ankle support.

The knee is always an area to watch.

Most basketballers now wear a high-cut boot to protect their ankle joints and prevent recurrent ankle injury. You need only to look at the National Basketball League in the United States and Australia to see that the majority of players wear high-cut boots. It's heartening to see this tendency filtering down into the minor leagues, setting the right example for young players.

Netball produces a fair number of girls with significant knee injuries.

'jumper's knee' which is a term like 'tennis elbow'. In such a case, it's wise to get several different diagnoses of anterior knee pain.

The pain might be caused by tenosynovitis or irritation on the undersurface of the kneecap. It could be a stress fracture to the patella, or perhaps inflammation to the outer covering of the patella. It could be any of a whole range of different conditions.

Osgood-Schlatters syndrome

One of these possibilities if Osgood-Schlatters syndrome (see p. 25). This is inflammation and possible separation of the patella tendon from the growth plate where the tendon attaches to part of the lower leg bone. The point of attachment is a protuberance known as a 'tuberosity'. There's a secondary growth plate in the tibia at this tuberosity. Varying degrees of inflammation occur, graded 1, 2, 3 or 4, depending on how far the area of bone has been pulled off the growth plate.

In children between 11 and 14, particularly the athletically involved, this can become a serious complaint because of the rapid pulling of the tendon when they run or jump.

Treatment

Treatment for the disorder used to involve immobilisation — putting the limb in a plaster cast for eight weeks. While this certainly settled the inflammation down, doctors found that the inflammation and consequent pain reappeared when the young athlete went back to normal activity.

The patient has to expect a period of pain and the doctor and patient just have to work together at this difficult time because it's a problem that takes a while to heal.

The treatment nowadays involves modifying the activities. The child is encouraged to participate but to limit this activity so as not to cause too much pain. After any such activity, apply ice to the affected area. The child is also given exercises to strengthen the quadriceps muscles.

Initially, anti-inflammatory medication may also be needed as it's quite a painful injury. The child may need a period of rest.

The aim is to build them back to enough activity to keep them happy and keep them going, but not too much to cause irritation to the injury.

Children suffering from this complaint should see the doctor every three to six months and should be re-examined after adolescence.

This particularly applies to those whose injury has involved the tendon being pulled off a fair way, often resulting in the need for an operation to screw the piece of bone back to a better position. Fortunately, only a small minority need such care.

However, they should not contemplate a return to their sport until the growth plate has finished growing. Then, if the bone is still off,

> **STOP**
> All injuries need prompt attention.

Screws, plates or pins should never be put across a growth plate.

> *Always be wary when knee pain persists, especially if it is affecting a child's ability to do schoolwork or daily physical activities besides sport.*

if it hasn't been attached properly, it can be screwed back in.

Screws, plates or pins should never be put across a growth plate. This effectively destroys the blood supply to that area and can cause premature closure of that growth plate.

OTHER KNEE INJURIES

Serious knee injuries, such as torn cartilages and damage to the joint surface, can cause severe knee pain. Always be wary when knee pain persists, especially if it is affecting a child's ability to do schoolwork or daily physical activities besides sport. If there is any clicking in the joint or if the joint catches when walking or running, then you should check for a condition called 'internal derangement'.

It could be a damaged meniscus, the consequence of which could be damage to the joint's cartilage. With the advent of arthroscopy, the complaint is not difficult to investigate and correct in its early stages.

Treatment

If there's a torn cartilage in an area where the doctor believes the blood supply is still available for healing, he might perform a meniscoplexy. This is the repair of a torn meniscus by sewing it back together. If the damage is more peripheral, towards the edge of the meniscus, the doctor might just remove the torn part, and the patient will get no further clicking or irritation of the joint.

However, if there's damage of the cartilage, a doctor may be able to pin it back into place to promote healing or, if the injury is more superficial, scrape off the damaged cartilage and smooth over the area.

A basketballer or netballer who lands heavily and has twisted his or her knee often feels no pain in the very early phases, even if the knee has been completely ruptured, because of the complexity and the unusual aspect of the nerve supply to the ligaments. Although they may feel a bit wonky and have to be taken off the court, they typically say, 'Oh, I've probably only just jarred my knee. I think I'm all right. It hasn't really started to swell or anything. I feel like going back on.'

This is now a very good time to make a manual examination of the knee. The injured child is not feeling a lot of pain so the muscles haven't gone tight to protect the knee. You may detect complete damage to the anterior cruciate ligament.

If the knee starts swelling rapidly, the swelling is due to bleeding into the joint. This is called a haemarthrosis and it means that something in the joint which has a blood supply, such as a ligament or a cartilage, is either fractured or torn and the blood is going into the joint. The result is a rapid collection of fluid over the next 30 minutes to 2 hours.

If the knee swells over perhaps 12 hours it's more likely to be a 'synovial effusion', that is, the lining of the joint has been irritated and this in turn

> *A basketballer or netballer who has twisted his or her knee often feels no pain in the very early phases.*

causes a build-up of fluid. The more information you have, the better, because you don't want to miss a major knee injury such as damage to an anterior cruciate ligament or a collateral ligament.

If a child has twisted a knee awkwardly, don't let that child back onto the field.

Observe the knee for the next few hours. If it rapidly swells, then you have a major knee injury. If it swells over the next 24 hours, you still may have a major knee problem. Use an appropriate medical centre for assessment, with X-rays to check for a fracture or an avulsion of the anterior cruciate ligament. If the athlete has difficulty putting weight on the knee, then suspect a serious injury.

Eventually, the child will end up with a normal knee again. But if the anterior cruciate ligament has been ruptured, then it's important to know that as early as possible. Reconstructing a knee can be tricky and it's something to avoid if at all possible.

Giving the surgeon and treating physicians as much information as possible about the injury allows for different treatment alternatives. The important thing is to get a knee injury seen early — in the first seven days.

If a medial or lateral collateral ligament is injured and there's undue delay in seeking medical treatment, by the time the doctor sees it the ligament may have retracted too much for the doctor to sew it back together. In the first few days, if a doctor has the option to repair it, the patient has a much better chance of a full recovery.

You can go to the GP rather than a specialist for that first assessment.

If the knee starts swelling rapidly, the swelling is due to bleeding into the joint.

Get a knee injury seen early — in the first seven days.

HELPFUL HINTS

- Check the court. Make sure the boundaries are well away from large immovable objects such as walls, posts, kiosks, tables and chairs.
- A warm-up is very important. Stretch the lower limbs: the muscles, the thighs, the hamstrings, the calves. Don't forget the lower back. Athletes doing these sports are using a lot of muscle groups so it is important to be flexible, particularly with the upper body.
- Wear the right shoes, particularly high-cut boots in basketball and possibly also in netball. Elbow and knee protectors give adequate protection for a heavy landing, particularly in volleyball. This also applies to basketball and netball. With outdoor courts, grazes to knees and elbows are very common.
- Be aware of the potential for injuries to the lower limbs, especially to the knee and its ligaments.
- The return to activities after injury should be graduated and involve a coordinated exercise program to strengthen the muscle groups involved.

CHAPTER 10

STRENGTH SPORTS: GYMNASTICS AND WEIGHTLIFTING

GYMNASTICS

Success in gymnastics calls for not only natural ability, but also long and gruelling practice sessions, sometimes twice a day, six days a week. The effects of such intense training should never be overlooked if serious, nagging injuries are to be avoided.

With surprisingly little publicity, Australia is headed for major success in gymnastics as can be seen with the results in Auckland and Barcelona. The sport is booming because of a recent, extensive recruiting drive in schools in all states. Girls are particularly attracted to gymnastics because of its disciplined grace and elegance and its close affinity with calisthenics.

Flexibility and strength are of paramount importance in gymnastics because of the very strenuous programs involved. In particular, considerable strength is needed in the lower body and the back, and in the development of good wrists and shoulders.

INJURIES

Routines on the uneven bars, floor routines, and jumping and tumbling, all put stress on the back, shoulders, upper limbs and extremities, knees and ankles.

Traumatic injuries — sprained ankles, wrists, elbows and knees — may occur, and, sometimes, dislocations.

Long-term problems can develop through overuse, because gymnasts become good at a very young age. It's possible for a 13- or 14-year-old to represent her/his country internationally. Such high expectations impose tremendous stress on these children and add to the amount of training they have to do. Overuse syndrome (fully discussed in Chapter 2) should and can be prevented.

It should be remembered that in sports such as weightlifting and gymnastics, more injuries happen in training than in actual competition. In training, children are practising difficult routines not quite perfected and may be fighting physical and mental fatigue, making them vulnerable to injury. Coaches and athletes must be on the alert for warning signs that an injury may be around the corner. They have to introduce new routines carefully until children build up the necessary strength.

The table on page 114 sets out injuries which occur in gymnastics.

AGE AND TRAINING IN GYMNASTICS

In a sense, some children start gymnastics in a play situation at the age of three or four. Then they just build up from there. Even at this early age, there's need for good coaching to ensure a sound progression of activities. It then all comes down to their capabilities physically, and, to some extent, emotionally, and to how much training they can tolerate.

I discussed in Chapter 1 how unrealistic training expectations can affect the emotional and psychological development of young athletes. Not only is their sport affected. So are their family life, their relationships with their peers at school and their mental calm and ability to cope with problems which are part and parcel of today's stressful lifestyle. Children can also be surprisingly well-tuned to any tensions in their home environment and any feelings of insecurity can have a major effect on their sporting performance.

All of these things are important and should be assessed carefully by the coach and parents if the child athlete is to progress to a high level of achievement at an early age. To do this, children need tremendous dedication, the iron-clad self-discipline to stick to a strenuous training program, a burning desire to succeed and the ability to cheerfully make tremendous sacrifices, especially in denying themselves a proper social life.

NUTRITIONAL PROBLEMS

Anorexia and bulimia are eating disorders that appear throughout the community. Anorexia is self-imposed starvation. Bulimia is episodes of binge eating followed by self-induced vomiting.

In activities where body shape and image are considerations, such as gymnastics, special care must be taken. These conditions need specialised medical and psychiatric attention. Coaches should be aware of some of the warning signs and take the appropriate action.

MENSTRUATION

Menstrual problems may also occur because intense exercise may delay or interfere with the regularity of menstruation and medical attention should be sought when this problem occurs.

CONSIDERATIONS FOR TRAINING

Coaches must be educated and sympathetic to the individual needs and abilities of their gymnasts, as well as being good communicators with

Unrealistic training expectations can affect the emotional and psychological development of young athletes.

In activities where body shape and image are considerations, such as gymnastics, special care must be taken.

athletes, parents and others who work with them.

Note that a sound program of physical preparation (warm up and cool down) is essential to prevent injury.

Spotting

'Spotting' means using the coach or assistant to help the gymnast complete a difficult or specific manoeuvre (such as on the beam, vault, rings). Children should not depend on spotting to perform skills at the beginner level but as the skill level rises, spotting becomes important.

The emphasis in beginner programs should be on encouraging the development of competent body management skills.

Coaches should be aware of the following points on spotting:

- When the skill level is low, the need for spotting is greatly reduced.
- In higher level programs, spotting becomes progressively more important.
- The spotting skills of the coach should match the performance level of the gymnast.
- Incompetent spotting is potentially dangerous. Spotting should never be used as a substitute for inadequate physical exercise, poor equipment, or poor technical preparation.

INJURIES WHICH OCCUR IN GYMNASTICS

MEDICAL CONDITION	LAY TERM	SYMPTONS AND SIGNS	PRINCIPLES OF MANAGEMENT	PRINCIPLES OF PREVENTION
Ligament sprain of ankle	Ankle sprain (twisted ankle)	Pain, tenderness, swelling, bruising around ankle	• RICE • Sports medicine as soon as possible	• Ankle exercises for balance • Taping as needed
Impingement of carpal bones	Wrist pain	Pain and tenderness to touch of back of wrist. Pain in weight-bearing (tumbling, vault, pommels, etc)	• Limit wrist work • Referral for tests by sports medicine practitioner	• Gradual increase in wrist work • Ice as necessary • Wrist guards • Strapping
Rotator cuff syndrome	Shoulder strain	Pain on lifting arm above shoulder level. Tenderness of shoulder to touch	• Restrict painful movement • Ice, stretch • Sports medicine referral	• Limit sudden increases in amount of shoulder work • Stretching
Stress fracture tibia or fibula	Stress fracture of shin or leg above ankle	Gradual appearance of pain and very local tenderness of bone in lower leg	• Rest from hard landings for up to six weeks • Medical referral for tests	• Gradual increase in leg work on floor, dismounts, etc
Spondylosis	Stress fracture of the spine	Low back pain especially on arching backwards or dismounts	• Restrict painful activities • Early referral to sports medicine practitioner	• Correct technique • Back strength and flexibility • Gradual increase in amount of back work

RECOMMENDATIONS FOR GYMNASTICS PARTICIPATION, TRAINING AND COMPETITION
(FROM THE AUSTRALIAN GYMNASTIC FEDERATION AND THE AUSTRALIAN SPORTS MEDICINE FEDERATION)

1 Coaches should have at least a Level 1 accreditation from coaching courses held by the Australian Gymnastic Federation.

2 Coaches, parents and teachers should have a minimum of Level 1 Accreditation from the National Sports Trainers Scheme.

3 Coaching programs must be individually tailored, taking into account:
- physical maturation level
- ability to learn new skills
- physical limitations, including injury.
- skill level
- degree of enthusiasm

4 Serious gymnasts should be screened by qualified sports medicine practitioners with expertise in gymastics for physical traits which may predispose them to injury.

5 Gymnasts need sound physical preparation, gradual development of skills and the acquisition of proper technique.

6 Coaches should encourage flexibility to the upper limit of the normal range of joint movement and not beyond — stretch and hold without pain. Coach- or teacher- assisted stretching is not recommended for beginner programs.

7 All complaints of pain, tenderness, limitation of movement or disability should be referred immediately to a qualified sports medicine professional. The spine, knees and wrists — the main areas of adolescent growth — should be watched.

8 Gymnastics coaches should be aware that a stress fracture of the spine is a particular hazard:
- It affects both sexes, especially in the 12 to 16 years age group.
- It is associated with hyperextension of the lower spine during impact.
- Never suddenly increase the number of times this movement is performed in training.
- Preventive strengthening programs decrease the chance of this injury occurring.

9 Training methods which reduce the number of times a child lands on competition surfaces are recommended. Use more mats, modified equipment or supplementary teaching stations.

10 Education of coaches and gymnasts in exercise, diet and weight control is recommended. Discuss eating disorders and manage them properly when identified. All female gymnasts need professional advice on menstrual disorders and should be referred to a medical practitioner if they have any concerns.

11 Although it is rare, delayed growth (measured against peers in non-gymnastic activities) should be referred for medical assessment.

12 Apparatus must be kept in good, safe, working condition, correctly erected and only used for its original purpose.

HORMONAL MANIPULATION

Hormonal manipulation is definitely rearing its head. In Australia it is not a major problem yet, but the dangers should be recognised now before it becomes prevalent.

Manipulating the suppression of hormone levels by chemical means is illegal but widespread, at least in Eastern European countries. If such techniques are available, some people will always be tempted to use them, no matter how irresponsible it is. The long-term effects of these drugs are not yet understood, but research work has started to investigate possible side-effects.

Most sports medicine doctors would have stories to relate from their casebooks. The best one from my experience was with a mother and daughter who came in to see me. The mother stunned me when she remarked that everything pointed towards her daughter being a champion gymnast over the next three or four years, if only her puberty could be delayed. 'The problem is to make her strong and small. I read in a magazine recently about boosting sporting performance by hormonal manipulation and I'm wondering if you can help.'

After recovering from my amazement, I tried to dissuade her. But they left clearly dissatisfied and very likely to continue their 'doctor shopping'.

While I don't believe this irresponsible attitude is prevalent in our society, I believe that it will be unless we are alert to the ever-increasing pressures for athletes to push themselves to the very limits of their physical abilities. Hormonal manipulation to boost performance will inevitably become a serious problem with people so blinded by the promise of sporting glory that they ignore the large question mark about long-term protection of their health.

Coaches should never force the gymnast to attempt a skill before the prerequisites are mastered.

Coaches should never force the gymnast to attempt a skill before the prerequisites are mastered.

WARM-UPS

A warm-up program is vital for both gymnastics and weightlifting. Adequate preparation of the particular muscle groups is necessary as both sports put muscles under so much stress.

I advise weightlifters to work on the wrists, the muscles around their elbows, shoulders, their lower back and the thigh muscles, the quadriceps and hamstrings, which are so important to stretch. I urge them to do a good 15 to 20 minutes warm-up before they start lifting.

Then they might use a broomstick to go through the routine of warming up their shoulders and going down into the squat position, just to go through the movements they are going to do before they start lifting a bar. The bar itself weighs 25 kg, so just starting with that is a fair weight.

It's important for gymnasts to stretch and flex the back, shoulders, wrists and elbows, as well as the knees, to properly prepare those muscles.

WEIGHTLIFTING

With any child starting basic weightlifting, good learning techniques are very important. Weightlifting can be started at the age of eight or nine, with the right coaching. This means starting with very light weights and perhaps using a junior bar. But in general, it means just learning the very fluid movements.

Weightlifting involves very precise and quite aesthetic movements. Learning how to do that takes a lot of time and skill. But once children learn that basic skill, they can build on the weights as they become stronger and bigger. I think one of the great attributes of coordinated weightlifting is that even children who have less strength than others of the same age can learn techniques such as lifting the bar correctly and then build on them as they get stronger.

Weightlifting has boomed in the last decade. Twelve years ago a schoolboy competition began in Melbourne with 500 boys. There are now 70,000 in Australia. One of the reasons is an excellent administrative program. Many physical education teachers realise that it's a great sport for all boys and girls in schools to get into because it tells them how to use weights correctly. Weightlifting can be very helpful for any sort of sport.

Clearly, a lot of the 70,000 children won't go on to do weightlifting into adulthood. There are simply not enough facilities. But there is a talent identification program to find the best ten in each division out of those 70,000 throughout Australia and then take them to the Australian Institute of Sport for specialised training. The special program there identifies the top 50 in Australia and these boys can be trained further. If we do this every year, we will produce world champions in the next ten years.

In many schools, like De La Salle in Melbourne, every boy in the school enters the schoolboy 'clean and jerk' program. The other thing which has been introduced is a schools' program which enables boys to compete against each other. We have an interschool program in Victoria which began in 1987. The three boys who were the inaugural champions were the most unlikely-looking boys — two big, lumbering-looking boys and one little fellow. Weightlifting is one of the few sports which allows a differentiation of body size and weight.

The little fellow was only 44 kg. No one thought he had any potential for football, basketball or cricket. He was just too small. But for weightlifting, in his division, he was number one in Victoria and number two in Australia. The two other boys were overweight and too slow for football. They won the heavy divisions in weightlifting.

Weightlifters must have a good ratio of height to body weight. In other words, they cannot be too tall. They must have a low centre of gravity. They must also have tremendous self-discipline and determination.

The major factor in good weightlifting is having an excellent technique. Australia has been

---

Weightlifting is one of the few sports which allows a differentiation of body size and weight.

Weightlifters must have a good ratio of height to body weight.

applauded internationally at a junior level for having the best technique in the world. Our excellent training programs and school programs enable us to teach children how to lift properly and then give them the opportunity to continue developing their skills.

FREE WEIGHTS AND WEIGHT TRAINING

There's no doubt that in any weight training program, the use of free weights is far superior to using those fantastic-looking machines in gyms. Free weights are now recognised as by far the most effective method of strength training. They put joints, such as the shoulders, elbow and wrist and also the spine, hips and knees, through the full range of movement. This is why so many coaches in football and other sports are now going back to using free weights in sports. I believe weight training has a big part to play in overall training for a wide range of sports — football, cricket, basketball, and track and field. The old adage was that runners, including those doing long-distance events, should never lift weights and should just go out there and run. But a back squat, for example, can be done with such power and force that it can build up tremendous strength in the muscles of the legs.

There is an important difference between power and strength. Strength is just the actual amount of force which can be generated. Power is force times velocity — strength and speed. Weightlifters are very powerful, whereas bodybuilders or powerlifters may be very strong. 'Powerlifting' is really the wrong word because powerlifters are not as powerful as Olympic weightlifters. They're strong but their movements are a lot slower. They do the dead lift, bench press and the squat, whereas weightlifting is a very dynamic sport, also involving the snatch and the clean and jerk.

Weightlifters lift the bar extremely quickly. In fact, few people realise that one of the fastest movements in any sport is the movement of the bar in one snatch from the floor to when it's secured overhead.

INJURIES

In terms of injuries, the things to look for are overuse injuries. When children begin to lift more regularly and increase the weights they are lifting, then they're going to get soreness in their wrists, shoulders and knees.

One of the biggest problems is anterior knee pain. This is pain caused by inflammation under the kneecap or the patella tendon, due to immense forces applied through the body when you squat down to lift up the weight and then hold it overhead.

The shoulders are also vulnerable because of the tremendous rotation in the snatch. The forces applied to the shoulder joint and the muscles around it can cause muscle strain and inflammation in the capsule joint. The

Free weights are the most effective method of strength training.

The things to look for are overuse injuries.

same can happen to the wrist.

Remember, weightlifters hold the bar with the wrist bent back. The amount of pressure applied to the wrist joint can cause irritation. Again, there may be discomfort without any really serious injury.

I haven't seen a torn major ligament in the knee in the 12 years I have been involved in weightlifting. I have seen a few meniscal tears and also several muscle ruptures, particularly involving the biceps (upper arm muscles) and quadriceps (the upper thigh and buttocks muscles). These usually involve the older athlete working with heavier weights.

Injuries are rare in the schoolboy and the junior programs. Many people comment to me that surely all weightlifters must have wrecked backs! But the fact is that very few have problems with their lower back, apart from having some soreness.

This again highlights the fact that, as with other sports, correct lifting is very important to strengthen the back muscles and those around the buttocks region. You can get some muscular strain in the lower back, but serious back injuries are not very common.

I would rate weightlifting as being one of the safest sports, if it is taught correctly and done sensibly. The program must be well run, children should have a good coach who has probably gone through one of the coaching programs run by the Australian Weightlifting Federation, and there should not be any overcrowding, which sometimes happens when there are people trying to lift weights all over the place. People might be dropping bars.

There should be good coordination and control by a senior person, such as a coach or trainer. This is one of the best ways to prevent accidents in a gymnasium. Accidents are usually caused by neglect and poor management. That's always a problem, as in any other sport, such as when high jumpers trys to jump too high. Prevention again comes back to the coach being in control. If you go to the major gyms, there's always close supervision. When you're training for competition, you're gradually pushed to your limit. But it's a limit at which your coach knows you're capable of performing.

> **GIRLS AND WEIGHTLIFTING**
>
> The success of the schoolboy and schoolgirl 'clean and jerk' competition shows that many girls are also interested in strength sports and in learning how to lift weights correctly: still not as much as boys, but the interest is growing.
>
> I personally believe that weightlifting lends itself more to males than females. But certainly girls can successfully learn the proper techniques and lift weights.

Correct lifting is very important to strengthen the back muscles and those around the buttocks region.

Accidents are usually caused by neglect and poor management.

If any blisters appear, they should always be looked after in training.

EQUIPMENT

Good weightlifting boots are not so important when children are just starting. A good pair of sandshoes is adequate. As children become more involved, it's advisable to get them a good pair of weightlifting boots with a strap around the top and a leather sole and a leather heel, to give them a little lift when they are going through the various movements. The extra support they give is well worth the price.

In weightlifting, you're allowed to have chalk on your hands and, if any blisters appear, they should always be looked after in training. You should always get to them promptly so they don't get infected because this could seriously interfere with the effectiveness of training and competition.

SUMMARY

One of the major issues in weightlifting, and also in gymnastics, is how we can best allow the body to recover from a gruelling training program. The prime treatment of overuse syndromes is prevention or early recognition.

These people train once or twice a day, six days a week, so we have to try to devise a method to help the body recover from these intense training programs. Sometimes, the training is far more intense than the competition!

We also have to help the body recover with massage, attention to vitamins and nutrition, hot baths and saunas, and a whole variety of treatments. This is a very important, and often overlooked, aspect of gymnastics and other sports involving intense training.

Ten Golden Rules for Children's Sport

1 Always remember that children are not little adults. Never let yourself be carried away with enthusiasm. It's wise to keep a commonsense perspective on your child's physical limits rather than expect him or her to achieve miracle performances.

2 Children should participate in a sport because they want to. They should not play because they are being pressured into it by their parents or school. If they are happy about doing a sport, they will be far less injury-prone.

3 An adequate warm-up is essential. It should be appropriate to the type of sport being undertaken. Always seek the advice of your school coach or a qualified sporting instructor if in doubt. Guesswork can be expensive in terms of your son or daughter's welfare. The frustration of being sidelined for weeks or months by a nagging injury can be prevented. There's also the disruption to family life that such an injury causes.

4 All children playing sport should have proper equipment. Possibly the most important part of all equipment is correct footwear. The proper equipment doesn't necessarily have to be the most costly, the one with a fancy name endorsing it. Good secondhand equipment is always preferable to a new item which is the wrong size, shape or is otherwise unsatisfactory. The importance of going to the trouble to make sure that all equipment is correctly fitted and matched to the size of the player cannot be overemphasised. For example, tennis racquets should be properly balanced to avoid wrist injuries. Children are better off with a mid-size racquet than an oversize head.

5 Carefully check the sporting venue for hazards. This applies to a football field and cricket ground — look for sprinkler heads, fences, seats and other obstructions too close to the boundary; a basketball court — look for the boundary too close to the wall; an outdoor netball court — look for broken asphalt, loose stones, and discarded drink containers and food litter. In horse riding, the course should always be checked, particularly near jumps, so that the rider is aware of possible hazards in case a horse shies at a jump. Knowing what's behind the bushes and trees or around the next bend could mean the difference (in that split second when you have to make a decision) between: (a) salvaging the situation, (b) being thrown and getting back on, and (c) head injuries.

6 Concentration is a must at all times. Always make sure children take a few minutes to close their eyes and prepare their minds before any sport. Mind and body are partners in any sporting event. Never let anyone play or ride when they are tired, unwell or just feeling out of sorts.

7 The first few hours following an injury are vital. That is the time to obtain appropriate treatment to avoid serious complications. Simple commonsense and basic first aid principles, particularly when dealing with soft tissue, muscle or joint injuries, can significantly aid recovery and prevent more significant secondary problems occurring.

8 Never return to a sport too soon after an injury. Always err on the side of caution, particularly with a head injury. Experience overwhelmingly shows that players who return too early are vulnerable to reinjury or will suffer a separate one. This is particularly true in contact sports such as football (all codes).

9 If it's an obvious injury, you should apply proper first aid. The best of all is RICE: rest, ice, compression, elevation. If you are still concerned about how the head, knee or shoulder injury is responding, then seek medical attention from a doctor. Do it promptly. Always accept medical advice about X-rays and being admitted to hospital for observation. Slow internal bleeding from a head injury can take time to show. If you had a smash in your car, you wouldn't keep driving it. Your body is much more important. Take good care of it. It's the only one you have been issued with. There are no trade-ins!

10 The best accident prevention device is you. Parents should be involved. Being there can make all the difference between a cut or a grazed elbow, and a broken arm. It doesn't take long for children to get enough confidence to do their own thing. Your son or daughter will also get the reassurance that you really care. So, make the time. It's one of the best investments you can possibly make.

THE PATTERN OF SPORTS IN AUSTRALIA

The pattern of sports in Australia is undergoing sweeping changes and, with that, the pattern of sports injuries is also changing. There's a strong trend in Australia for parents and children to go for sports which have an international flavour and representation. That's why we're seeing, to some extent, a decline in the time-honoured sports in this country — cricket and football. Even Rugby is limited to Commonwealth countries and France. Netball's world championships are played by several countries, but this also has its limitations.

Soccer, on the other hand, is universal. The World Cup stands supreme.

Basketball is also an international sport. Australian Rules football and Rugby can be very violent sports. Parents are understandably concerned. For example, head injuries and serious injuries to knees are common, which isn't good for the sport. Basketball and soccer tend to be far less violent.

If our community is trying to encourage life-long physical activity, we need to pay more careful attention to offering suitable games and recreations to school children. It is also sensible to encourage sports which people can play all their lives, so they can improve and enjoy their skills.

GLOSSARY

Achilles-tendonitis: Inflammation of the tendon of the calf muscle at the back of the leg.
Antagonists: Muscles that produce an opposition movement at a joint.
Anterior cruciate ligament: The main internal ligament of the knee.
Anthropometric measurements: A scientific method of classifying people into body types so they can be better matched to sports to enhance performance and minimise injury. For example, tall and agile for basketball, short and muscular for weightlifting.
Arthrogram: A test involving injecting dye into a joint to assess damage to the surface, giving information an X-ray cannot provide.
Arthroscopy: A simple operation, under anaesthetic, where a small hole is made in the joint in which is inserted a tiny telescope-like instrument with a light source. Doctors can see the internal aspects of the joint, be it the knee, shoulder, ankle or wrist joint. Through other small holes made in the joint, instruments can be inserted and investigative procedures performed. This avoids the need to make a large incision to open the joint to perform such procedures.
Aseptic avascular necrosis: Death to an area of tissue because of lack of blood — not due to an infection.
Avascular: Without a blood supply.
Avulsion injury: When either a ligament or a tendon, instead of rupturing when the force is applied, tends to pull off where it's attached to the bone. This is because a tendon or ligament is stronger than the bone, usually in the area where the tendon is attached.
Biceps: A double-bellied flexor muscle in the upper arm.
Biomechanical studies: Studies about the movement of the body and the forces involved to produce those movements.
Bursa: The sac which is bathing area with fluid around the common tendon group.
Capital femoral epiphysis: Growth plate head in the thigh bone.

Cartilage: Connective tissue lining part of a joint.
Closed injuries: No open cuts but possible internal bruising or bleeding. A closed head injury can be quite serious.
Collagenous tissues: These include ligaments and capsules. The main purpose of a warm-up is to raise both the general body and the deep muscle temperatures and to stretch the muscles and collagenous tissues to promote greater flexibility.
Collateral ligaments: A ligament supporting either side of a joint. They are not just at the knee, but also at the elbow and other joints.
Concussion: A closed head injury — usually not a subarachnoid nor a subdural, which are the big problems. But there is still bruising and damage to some part of the brain tissue, which may be serious.
Contusion: A bruise involving slight bleeding into the tissues while the skin remains unbroken.
Corticosteroid: A combination of cortisone and a steroid used as an effective anti-inflammatory treatment.
Cystic lesions: Cyst formation in a tissue.
Developmental lesions: Problems which occur during the growth period.
Diathermy: Electrical method of producing heat.
Differential diagnosis: Different causes of a particular problem or symptom. For example, the differential diagnosis of pain in a joint could be a tumour or a whole range of other possibilities.
Divot: An area where there's been an excavation of bone or tissue.
Ectoderm: A lean and tall body type.
Endoderm: A fat and squat body type.
Epiphysis: A growth centre of a bone.
Extensor muscle: One which, on contraction, extends or straightens a part.
Femoral head: The head of the thigh bone.
Femur: The thigh bone.
Fibula: The outer of the two bones forming the lower leg.
Genetic predisposition: An inherited weakness in a person's physical make-up which can mean

they are prone to certain injuries.
Glue ears: Condition in which thick fluid collects behind the eardrum in the middle ear. It's called a middle ear infection because the fluid doesn't drain away into the back of the throat.
Gluteal: Pertaining to the buttocks.
Golfer's elbow: Painful inflammation of the inner aspect of the elbow joint, originally and commonly seen in golfers because of the stress to this area when swinging a golf club. This condition is known as 'medial epicondylitis'.
Growth centres: Embryonic areas in bone from which growth is initiated.
Growth plates: Another name for growth centres.
Haemarthrosis: Bleeding into a joint cavity, usually rapid, which may indicate: (a) significant damage to some internal structure of the joint, such as a major ligament; (b) a fracture involving the joint; (c) a torn meniscus in a knee joint. Anything which has a good blood supply can bleed into a joint.
Haematoma: A swelling filled with blood. The cause is usually bleeding within the muscle due to damage of the muscle fibres and the small blood vessels within the tissues.
Haemostasis: Stopping bleeding.
Hyperextension: Straightening a joint beyond the normal range.
Hyperthermia: High body temperature.
Hypothermia: Low body temperature.
Iliotibial band: The band of collagenous tissue running on the outer side of the thigh from the hip to the tibia.
Intra-articular fracture: An injury to the joint surface cartilage and the maturing bone beneath the surface. Invariably, such a fracture will require an operative procedure for proper re-establishment of a smooth joint surface.
Inversion injury: Common in racquet sports and football, this is the most common ankle sprain, in which the foot turns in and under, damaging the outer or lateral ligament.
Isokinetic aspect of muscles: The strength of a muscle through an accommodating force, that is, the greater the pressure applied, the greater the resistance.
Isometric muscle strength: The strength of a muscle against an immovable force. For example, applying force through a muscle by leaning against a wall.
Isotonic muscle strength: The strength of a muscle as it's moving a weight against a variable resistance. The resistance becomes greater as it's lifted higher against gravity.
Kinesiology: The study of the motion of joints.
Kohler's syndrome: See *Osteochondroses*.
Kyphosis: A rounding deformity of the thoracic spine.
Lateral epicondylitis: The classic description of pain over the outer or lateral aspect of the elbow joint. This condition is also called Tennis Elbow. While this is common in many sports, it gained its name because it was very common in tennis players. It is caused by the forces generated by the backhand.
Medial epicondylitis: See *Golfer's elbow*.
Meniscoplexy: The repair of a torn cartilage by sewing it back. This is only possible if the doctor believes the blood supply is still sufficient for healing.
Meniscus: Cartilage disc in the knee joint.
Mesoderm: A muscular body type.
Myositis ossificans: Calcification of a haematoma — a swelling filled with blood.
Myotatic reflex: A muscle-protective mechanism which is invoked during a stretching manoeuvre.
Navicular bone: Small bone in the foot on the inner or medial side.
Neuromuscular coordination: The coordination of movement involving the nervous and muscular systems.
Open injuries: An open fracture means that the fracture is exposed to the external environment. This means that there's been a laceration through the skin and the wound may be down to the bone. The bone, if broken, is exposed. This used to be called a 'compound' fracture.
Osgood-Schlatter's syndrome: Inflammation and possible separation of the growth plate where the patella tendon attaches to the upper tibia.
Osteochondritis: An inflammation of bone and cartilage.
Osteochondritis dissecans: A defect in the joint-bone cartilage of any synovial joint — knee, wrist, elbow, ankle. An X-ray of the area looks like a divot out of the joint surface.
Osteochondromas: Tumour involving bone and cartilage.
Osteochondrosis: An inflammatory process

involving both the cartilage and the bone in an area such as the femoral head (the head of the thigh bone) or the navicular one of the foot. Other osteochondroses occur in the vertebral bodies of the spine and during adolescence and account for postural deformities such as round back (kyphosis).
Overuse syndrome: An injury due to using an area excessively over a long period.
Patella tendon: The tendon of the thigh muscle.
Pathological fractures: A break in a bone which has something wrong with it already, such as a tumour.
Pedicle: A small stalk or stalk-like support, particularly a bony process of the spinal column.
Plantar fascia: The band of tissue which runs across the sole of the foot from the front of the heel bone to the bases of all of the toes. This is a very important ligament because it helps maintain the arches of the foot and prevents the forebones of the foot from spreading out, particularly when taking weight on the foot.
Proprioceptor: One of the body's key sensory receptors responsive to internal stimuli from muscles, joints and tendons.
Quadriceps: Thigh muscles.
RICE: An abbreviation standing for rest, ice, compression and elevation in treating sports injuries.
Rotator cuff syndrome: Inflammation of a tendon or a common group of tendons which produce the rotatory movements of the arm at the shoulder joint. This is a common problem with players of racquet sports, basketballers and swimmers.
Round back: Kyphosis — a rounding of the spine, usually in the thoracic region. One of the most common causes is Scheuermann's disease in childhood or early adolescence.
Scheuermann's disease: Inflammation of the cartilage lining the vertebral bodies, usually in the thoracic spine.
Sever's disease: A pulling of the insertion of the tendo-Achilles on the back of the heel bone.
Sorbathane™: A trademarked artificial shock-absorbent substance used extensively in the inner soles of running shoes.
Subarachnoid haemorrhage: Serious arterial bleeding due to the bursting of an artery, resulting in a rapid deterioration in the injured player's condition.
Subdural haemorrhage: Another type of potentially life-threatening brain haemorrhage. A subdural haemorrhage is due to a venous bleed between two layers covering the brain.
Subluxations: The incomplete dislocation of a joint.
Subtalar joint: Just below the ankle joint.
Synovial effusion: Fluid collecting in a joint due to an increased production of lubricant fluid by the synovium. Overproduction can be caused by a number of factors including a loose body in the joint, a tear in the meniscus or irritation of the synovium due to arthritis. This leads to an effusion — a swelling.
Synovial joint: A joint lined by synovium. These are usually the major joints of the body: the shoulder, the elbow, the knee, the ankle. Synovial joints include the small joints in fingers.
Synovium: The inner lining under the capsule beneath the capsule joint.
Tarsal-navicular bone: A key bone in the foot.
Tendo-Achilles: The large tendon of the calf muscle running down the back of the lower leg attaching to the heel bone.
Tendonitis: An inflammation of the tendon usually involving the outer sheath. It can be acute, meaning it can come on very rapidly because of overstress, or it can come on slowly because of overuse. It's commonly seen in children and young adolescents involved in long-distance running or in the upper arms, shoulders or elbows of pitchers or bowlers who have thrown the ball too long or too hard.
Tennis elbow: The classic description of pain over the outer, or lateral, aspect of the elbow joint. See *Lateral epicondylitis*.
Tenosynovitis: Inflammation affecting a tendon sheath. The condition may be either acute or chronic. Any injury to a tendon sheath may result in tenosynovitis. The symptoms are pain and swelling along the course of the tendon. The usual treatment is RICE: rest, ice, compression and elevation.
Tibia: The major bone in the lower part of the leg between the knee and the ankle.
Trauma: Any injury.
Tympanic membrane: The eardrum.
Vulva: The external area around the vagina.

INDEX

abrasions 56
Achilles tendon (tendo-Achilles) 124
   exercise 93
   injury 40–1, 81, 97, 98
Achilles-tendonitis 123
acromioclavicular joint 50
age pattern of sport 15
alcohol 73
ankle
   injuries 81, 89, 91–2, 93
   pads 90
   sprains 91–2, 94–7, 114
   straps 71–2
anorexia 113
antagonists 123
anterior cruciate ligament 110, 123
anterior knee pain 118
anthropometric measurements 123
arena *see* playing area
arm injuries 81, 99
arthogra 26
arthroscopy 26, 51–2, 123
aseptic avascular necrosis 123
aspirin 19
athletics 29–43
athrogram 123
Australian Sports Medicine Federation 106
Australian Sports Trainers Association 106
avascular 123
avulsion injury 21–2, 23, 97, 123

back assessment 93
badminton 91–105
ball 58
baseball 58–67
basketball 105, 106–11
batting gloves 59
bells, cycle 77–8
biceps 35, 123
bicycle riding 77–87
bicycles 77–8
biomechanical studies 123
blisters 42
blood supply 18, 23
Blu-Tac ear plugs 70
BMX bike riding 77–87
BMX clubs 82
bone scan 65
bones 20–8
   cysts 27
   damage 62
   developmental lesions 27
   fracture *see* fractures
   osteochondroses 23–6
   overuse syndromes 22–3
   tumours 27
boogie boards 72
boots *see* footwear
boundary lines 61
bowling guidelines 65–6
boxing 86

braces 103
brain injury *see* head injuries
bras 59
breast protection 59
breaststroker's knee 74
breathing difficulties 83
bruises 61–2
buddy system in surfing 71
bulimia 113
burnout 10
bursa 123
bursitis 37

capital femoral epiphysis 123
car seat belts 79
carbohydrate 12, 13
cartilage 109–10, 123
chest injuries 54–5
choosing a sport 7–8
climatic conditions 30–1
closed injuries 123
collagenous tissues 123
collapse 83
collarbone fracture 81
collateral ligaments 123
communication problems 10
compression (*see also* RICE) 16
concentration 121–2
concussion 85–7, 123
contusion 123
corticosteroid 123
cortisone injections 99
courts *see* playing area
cramps 71
crash-helmets *see* helmets
cricket 58–67
cuts 56
Cybex 91
cycling 77–87
cyst 27
cystic lesions 123

deformity 20–1, 25
dehydration 32, 60
developmental lesions 27
diathermy 123
diet *see* food
differential diagnosis 123
dilating pupils 83
dislocations
   finger 48–9
   shoulder 49–50
divot 123
doctor, when to see 16–18
double vision 83
drinks break 60
driving safety 79

ear-drops 70
ear drum 70
ear infections 69–70, 74, 76
ear plugs 70
ectoderm 123
elbow
   epicondylitis 100–4
   exercise 93
   injuries 64, 81

pads 88, 111
pain 100
   protectors 78–9
elevation (*see also* RICE) 16
endoderm 123
endurance swimming 72
epicondylitis 100–3, 124
epiphysis 21, 123
equipment (*see also* protective equipment) 14–15, 121
   bat and ball games 67
   football 57
   swimming 70–1
   water sports 76
   weightlifting 120
exercises (*see also* warm-up)
   ankle 92–3
   racquet sports 104
   trunk-strengthening 75
extensor muscle 123
eye-drops 69, 70
eyes
   dilating pupils 83
   infections 69, 76
   injuries 104–5
   irritated 74

faceguard 59
fall safety 90
fatigue 10
femoral head 123
femur 123
fibula 123
field hockey 58–67
finger dislocations 48–9
first aid course 6
flags, cycle 77–8
floors, slippery 107
fluid intake 60
food 12–14
   before the game 12–13
   during the game 14–15
   after the game 14
foot injuries
   blisters 42
   inversion injury 91
   long-distance running 41–2
   skiing 89
   stress fractures 39
football 44–57
footwear 121
   bat and ball games 58, 67
   football 45, 57
   netball and basketball 107–8, 111
   racquet sports 91, 93
   running 33, 43
   skiing 89
   weightlifting 119–20
forearm fracture 81
fractures (*see also* stress fractures)
   arm 81, 88
   collarbone 81
   intra-articular 21
   pathological 27
   result of trauma 15
   ribs 54

tibia 89
free weights 118
function loss 18

genetic predisposition 123
gloves, batting 59
glucose 13
glue ears 69, 123
gluteal 123
glycogen 12
goal posts 44
goggles 69, 105
golfer's elbow (medial epicondylitis) 100, 123
groin
   injuries 81
   protectors 59
grommets 70
growth centres 20–1, 123
growth spurts 6–7, 68
gymnastics 112–16

haemarthrosis 110, 123
haematoma 46, 48, 123
haemostasis 123
hamstring injury 82
head injuries 53, 82–7, 90
headache 83
heel injuries 97–9
helmets
   bat and ball games 58
   boxing 86
   cycling 78, 79, 86, 90
   horse-riding 87
hepatitis B 56
high jump 31
hip
   iliotibial band injury 37
   osteochondrosis 24
hockey 58–67
home environment 10
hormonal manipulation 116
horse riding 86, 87–8
horses 88
hot weather 31
humid weather 31
hyperextension 123
hyperthermia 123
hypothermia 73–4, 123

ice (*see also* RICE) 16
   massage 36, 38
ice skating 90
iliotibial band 123
   exercise 38
   injury 37–8
IncrediBall 58
infections 18, 56
inflammation
   arm muscles 99, 100
   foot 41–2
   patella tendon 39, 109
inflammatory cells 18
insoles 59
insulin 13
internal derangement 110
internal injury 55

126   The Children's Sports Injuries Handbook

international sports 105
intra-articular fracture 21, 123
inversion injury 91, 124
isokinetic aspect of muscles 124
isometric muscle strength 93, 124
isotonic muscle strength 93, 124

joint injuries (*see also* ankle; elbow; knee; ligament injuries; shoulder)
  bat and ball sports 62
  finger 48–9
  football 48–52
  hip 24, 37
  osteochondritis dessicans 25–6
  seeing a doctor 16
jump
  high 31
  long 30–1
  muscle injuries 35
'jumper's knee' 108

kinesiology 124
knee (*see also* patella tendon)
  bandages 45
  iliotibial band injury 38
  injuries 50–2, 74, 81, 89, 108–11
  pads 88, 107, 111
  pain 24, 109–10, 118
  protectors 78–9
Kohler's syndrome 25
kyphosis 124

landing pits 43
  high jump 31
  long jump 30
lateral epicondylitis 100–3, 124
leg (*see also* Achilles tendon; knee; thigh)
  fracture 88
  stress fractures 39, 114
Legg-Perthes syndrome 24
ligament injuries (*see also* avulsion injury) 52, 74, 76
limp 24
Little Leaguer's Elbow 64
long-distance running 29, 32–3, 41–2
long jump 30–1

management 9–11
  athletics 30–1
  gymnastics 114
marathons 32
massage, ice 36, 38
mattresses 31
maturation 6–7
meals *see* food
medial epicondylitis (golfer's elbow) 100, 123
memory loss 53
meniscoplexy 110, 124
meniscus 50, 110, 124
menstrual problems 113
mesoderm 124
minerals 12
minimising injury 11
motivation 10
muscles (*see also* avulsion injury)
  injuries 34–7, 46–8, 82
  strains 68–9, 76
  testing 92–3
  tissue development 6

myositis ossificans 48, 124
mytatic reflex 124

navicular bone 124
net practice 59–60
netball 106–11
neuromuscular coordination 124
night cycling 79
non-stretch tape 14–15, 52
nutrients 18
nutrition 12–14, 113

open injuries 124
Osgood-Schlatter's syndrome 25, 109, 124
osteochondritis 124
osteochondritis dessicans 25–6, 124
osteochondromas 124
osteochondroses 23–6, 124
otitis externa 74
overstressed muscles 34–5
overuse injuries 15, 22–23, 124
  bat and ball games 67
  gymnastics 112
  running 29
  weightlifting 118
oxygen 18

pads, protective *see* protective equipment
pain
  elbow 99–100
  knee 24, 109–10, 118
  overuse syndromes 22–3
  seeing a doctor 16
  wrist 114, 118
parental involvement 80, 107, 122
patella femoral joint 74, 81
patella tendon 109, 124
  inflammation 39, 88
pathological fractures 27, 124
pedicle 124
plantar fascia 124
playing area 121
  athletics 30
  bat and ball games 61
  cycling 90
  football 44, 57
  netball and basketball 107, 111
pole vault 31
postural deformities 25
power 118
pre-game meal 12
proprioception 14
proprioceptor 14
protective equipment (*see also* helmets)
  bat and ball sports 58–9
  cycling 78–9, 90
  football 45
  horse-riding 88
  ice skating 90
  netball and basketball 107, 111
protein 12
pupils, dilating 83

quadriceps 124

racquet sports 91–105
racquets 103
recovery time 18
Red Cross 6

reflective tape 79
rehydration stations 32
respiratory difficulties 83
rest (*see also* RICE) 16
resuming sport after injury 18–19
ribs, fractured 54
RICE 16–17, 48, 124
riding 86, 87–8
rollerblading 86
rotator cuff
  inflammation 99
  lesion 63
  syundrome 114, 124
round back 124
rubber pontoons 31
rules
  bat and ball games 61, 67
  football 46, 57
running 29, 34–40
  long-distance 29, 32–3, 41–2

safety vests 73, 76
sailing 72–3
salt tablets 12
Scheuermann's disease 25, 124
seat belts 79
Sever's disease 97, 124
shinpads 59
shoes *see* footwear
shoulder
  dislocation 49–50
  exercise 93
  injuries 63–4, 74, 99
  strain 114
skateboard riding 81, 82, 86
skating 89–90
skeleton 20–8
'ski stock thumb' 89
skiing 88–9, 90
skin injury 56
slipped epiphysis 21
snow-skiing 88–9
soccer 105
softball 58–67
Sorbathane 59, 67, 124
'spearing' 53–4
spine
  injuries 53
  osteochondrosis 25
  stress fractures 64–5, 114
spleen damage 54
spondylosis 114
sprains, ankle 91–2, 94–7, 114
sprinting injuries 35
squash 91–105
St John Ambulance 6
strapping 14
street safety 80
strength 118
stress 10
stress fractures 15
  athletics 39–40
  bat and ball games 65
  diagnosing 40
  gymnastics 114
stretching exercises 9
  bat and ball games 60
  thigh muscles 36
subarachnoid haemorrhage 124
subdural haemorrhage 124
subluxations 124
subtalar joint 124
sugar 12, 13
supraspinatus tendonitis 74
surfboards 71–2

surfing 71–2
sweat 12, 107
swimmer's ear 74
swimmer's shoulder 74
swimming 68–71
  endurance 72
synovial effusion 110, 124
synovial joint 124
synovium 51, 124

tackling 53
tape, non-stretch 14–15, 52
tarsal-navicular bone 124
temperature
  hyperthermia 123
  hypothermia 73–4, 123
tendo-Achilles *see* Achilles tendon
tendonitis 23, 124
tendons *see* Achilles tendon; avulsion injury; patella tendon
tennis 91–105
tennis elbow 99–100, 125
tenosynovitis 100, 125
thigh
  iliotibial band injury 37–8
  injury 82
  stretching exercises 36
thumb injury 89
tibia 125
  fracture 89
track *see* playing area
track sports *see* athletics
traction injury 100
training
  bat and ball games 59–60
  football 45–6, 57
  gymnastics 112–14, 113–14, 115
  netball and basketball 106
  water-skiing 72
  water sports 76
  weightlifting 120
trauma injuries 15, 125
triceps 35
trunk-strengthening exercises 75
tuberosity 109
tumours, bone 27
tympanic membrane 125

ulna collateral ligament 89

visors 59
vitamins 12
vulva 125

warm-up (*see also* exercises) 8, 121
  bat and ball games 60–1, 65
  gymnastics 116
  netball and basketball 111
  racquet sports 93–4
  running 37, 43
  skateboarding 82
  water sports 76
water 32, 60
water-skiing 72–3
water sports 68–75
weather 30–1, 90
weightlifting 116–20
wet weather 30
wounds 56
wrist
  pain 114, 118
  straps 72

QUICK-FIND INJURY INDEX

Use this quick-find index for the appropriate treatment for specific injuries.

Achilles tendon 40
ankle sprains 94–6, 114
avulsion injuries 97

blisters 42
bone injuries 23–7, 62
bruising 61–2

chest injuries 55
concussion 85–7

dislocations
   finger 48–9
   shoulder 49–50

ear infections 70, 74
elbow injuries 64, 101
eye infections 69, 74

finger dislocation 48–9
foot injuries 41–2
fractures 40, 65, 114
function loss 18

head injuries 53, 83, 85–7
heel injuries 98
hip injuries 24

infection 18

joint injuries 16, 62
   ankle 94–6, 114
   elbow 64, 101
   finger 48–9
   hip 24
   knee 39, 40, 51–2, 74, 108, 109, 110–11
   shoulder 49–50, 63–4, 74, 99, 114

knee injuries 39, 40, 51–2, 74, 108, 109, 110–11

leg injuries 40, 114
limp 24

muscle injuries 23, 35–6, 47–8, 69

pain 16

shoulder injuries 49–50, 63–4, 74, 99, 114
spinal injuries 25, 54, 114
sprain, ankle 94–6, 114
stress fractures 40, 65, 114

tendon injuries 40
thigh injuries 38

wounds 56
wrist strain 114